MW00718306

Conquering Your Mountains

Veronica Cox

Conquering Your Mountains

Published by Leading Through Living Community, LLC

Cover credits: Background image by Koan, Photo by Joshe Martin, Design by Lynita Mitchell-Blackwell

Edited by Lynita Mitchell-Blackwell

Assistant Editors: David Good, Solomon J. Herbert, Janice Deneise Nash, Christian Edwards, Thurgood Marshall Jones, Jr.

Scripture quotations are from the Holy Bible, King James Version (KJV), www.Bible.com.

For Information, Contact:
Leading Through Living Community, LLC
6790 Broad Street Suite 300
Douglasville, GA 30135

ISBN-13: 978-0-9891457-6-3

SPECIAL DEDICATION

To my dearest friend, Harold Newton, you showed me the beauty of how a person truly gives from their heart - unconditional love was what you showed me; the core of your soul was so sweet and caring, so kind and pure. You were a true giver - of yourself and of your love to all you met. All who crossed your path were touched by your expressions of love. I have not met another angel like you. I will always love you Harold. I constantly thank God for bringing you into my life; you enriched me as a person and I am truly blessed to have known you. If I had never known I was loved, your actions would have made it known to me. Because of you, I now know what true love is. Thank you. Rest in peace my dear sweet friend... rest in peace.

NOTE FROM THE AUTHOR

The names of the men with whom I had relationships have been changed.

ACKNOWLEGMENTS

I would like to first thank my Lord and Savior Jesus Christ. If it was not for Him, there would be no me.

Thank you Phillis E. Cox, my beloved sister and sweet soul.

Bobbie Cox, who has shown me you can do anything you can put your mind to - RIP my dear sister.

My niece and nephew, Christian & Ashley Edwards; they have brought joy to my life, thank you.

My niece Georgia Robinson, she is truly a sweet spirit and an angel sent from heaven.

My God children: William Nash, you are the apple of my eye; and Alison Nash, may you rest in peace my sweet angel, I will love you forever.

To my family, thank you for being YOU!

To my LA family, Dorothy and Wade Odom, Sally and Arthur May: your love and support is appreciated.

Thanks to my sweet and dear cousin Arcola Green Morris for having such a beautiful spirit.

Icilda D. Orr, thanks for over 35 years of true friendship, your support has been priceless. Thank you for being a listening ear! You were there for me when I needed you and I appreciate that.

My friend I have known for at least 40 years - thank you Debbie Kicklighter!

To Pat Tobin of Tobin & Associates for giving me the opportunity to work with her in her PR Firm; rest in peace Pat.

Patricia Herbert, my classmate in make-up school, a beautiful soul and person; RIP Pat.

My friend, Leon Newton, who did not let anything stop him or get in the way of his success.

To all my instructors at the Elegant International, Inc., Academy of Professional Makeup for encouraging me and making me feel that my work was great.

Many thanks to The Masquers Club for being there when I needed you and giving me an opportunity to gain so much meaningful professional experience in backstage, onstage, and make up artistry for Theater.

Afram House Cosmetics for giving me my first job in the beauty industry.

To Ruth Nao Towns, my first roommate and one of the nicest people that you could ever meet.

Thank you Bob and Juanita Guess for selling me my first business, Rest in peace Bob.

Thank you to the San Francisco Urban League, through which I was able to work with Afram House Cosmetics, which was my introduction to the makeup industry.

Ervin Brownstein, a kind person who was in the right place at the right time when I needed him. RIP Ervin.

Patrice Coleman - for being there for me when I needed you, for assisting me in becoming a member of the Union Local 798 Makeup & Hair, and for helping me get my first job with Tyler Perry. Thank you so much!!!

Delilah Rashell Williams, for giving me a chance to work with her on her stage plays. Thank you Delilah!

Heartfelt thanks goes to Vanessa Williams for encouraging me to get started on this book.

To my Higher Living Christian Church family, thanks for just being loving and caring - I love you all.

My beloved Pastor, Andre' Landers, for encouraging and giving me my spiritual guidance, support and covering that has helped me on my journey in more ways than I can ever express.

To William H.D. Hornaday, the former pastor of Founder's Church of Religious Science in LA, thank you for helping me become aware of the power of the mind. Rest n peace, Dr. Bill.

To my San Francisco family, our time together was the highlight of my life; you know who you are.

To my principle, E.J. Oliver, the dad of us all at Fairfield Industrial High School, you were the best of the best; may your soul rest in peace.

To my graduating class, the class of 1962 of Fairfield Industrial High School, I am glad to have been a part of such a great legacy of achievers.

FOREWORD

The old adage is true: you can't judge a book by its cover.

Veronica Cox is the perfect example of this sage advice. Having come out of the Civil Rights Movement myself, I have always admired and respected "Ronnie", as she is affectionately known, since I first met her nearly 40 years ago.

Ronnie was a standout student at a film industry makeup school in Los Angeles, preparing for her behind-the-scenes career in movies and television. What struck me about her back then was that with her striking good looks and her trademark white gardenia in her hair, she could have actually pursued her calling in front of the cameras. But she was somewhat shy and unpretentious, and perhaps I thought, maybe not up to the challenges of the Hollywood lifestyle. Little did I know then that beneath this calm and beautiful exterior was a fighter who was up to any challenge: a strong and powerful sister who doesn't know the meaning of the word 'quit'.

As our lifelong friendship evolved, I learned many things about Ronnie – for instance, that as a teenager she had marched with Dr. Martin Luther King, Jr. in Birmingham. More importantly, I learned many things *from* Ronnie, such as how to dream big and keep your dream alive; how to face adversity with a positive outlook; and perhaps most of all, the idea that giving up on what you believe in your heart is right is not an option.

Now that Ronnie has embarked on the 'Public Speaking and Storytelling' chapter of her life, I know that she will win over many fans with her passion and spiritual wisdom, which are guaranteed to have a positive and uplifting impact on their lives; and this outstanding book will only serve to hasten that process.

Solomon J. Herbert
Publisher, Journalist and Photographer

MY GIFT TO YOU

If anyone has experienced a life of pain, grief, loss, trauma, and drama, it is me. I am the first to say that it is not easy to forget hurtful things that have deeply pierced the core of one's being. Hurt and pain have a way of leaving long-lasting scars on us and in us. These "scars" or memories affect how we see ourselves and the world around us, and affect every relational encounter we have going forward. However, we have the power to change that!

By sharing my life experiences of trial, tragedy, and triumph, I hope to offer you encouragement through the tough times in your life, to inspire you to see the light at the end of the tunnel, to give you hope that "trouble don't last always" and that "this too shall pass." No matter what circumstances or situations have come against you to try to prevent, block, or deter God's plan from manifesting in your life; the words from my heart to yours are, "Hold on to your faith, no matter what." You must have faith and with faith, joy will come.

TABLE OF CONTENTS

PREFACE

In the journey of life, you are always in some phase of a storm: either going into a storm, in the midst of a storm, or coming out of a storm. Each storm makes you stronger and prepares you to handle the next one with more courage, understanding and strength.

Storms are metaphorical challenges. Our challenges come to teach us something about ourselves and others, and each transition although painful is for our benefit. In other words, **our pain has a purpose.**

Storms have finite periods, but can feel infinite. Some last a short season and others seem to endure for a lifetime. However, the pain that we experience is not intended to hurt or damage us, but to help and build us up. This statement sounds like a bit of a contradiction, but it is not. Our pain actually serves various purposes: to mold, develop, and pull out "the best parts of us" which are often deep down inside and buried under fear, doubt, or some area of unbelief. Pain gives us a signal to the areas within us that require attention, healing, or elimination. It pushes us toward manifestation of our greatest selves - our God nature.

While going through a storm, we must remain focused on the intended outcome and the truth about what is really happening. No matter how hard it may seem, how low we may feel, or how powerless we appear against our adversities and adversaries in life; these negative feelings usually are accompanied by distorted perceptions about ourselves and what is truly happening in our lives. The truth is that troubles and trials come into our lives to make us stronger, solidify our faith, and position us to be who we REALLY are - great and powerful children of God.

Our life experiences have a way of lying to us. We hear negative messages and go through traumatic experiences at the hands of others that make us fearful of our futures and doubt our ability to succeed. These personal violations of trust make us doubt our value and worth in general and also affect the way we think about ourselves and others. Our thinking then negatively affects our hopes, aspirations, and motivations to live our dreams. Yet in spite of all the negative images and messaging that drain us mentally, emotionally, and sometimes even physically; we are not the sum total of our experiences.

We are created by The Almighty for greatness, to be a reflection of greatness: a reflection of God Himself on the earth. We were created to demonstrate greatness in everything that we do by using our gifts and talents to make the world a better place. That means that at any given moment we may turn away from the negative programming and experiences we previously encountered and choose to live a life of greatness.

God has a good plan for all of His children, a plan to bless us, bring us to a place of seeing our deepest hopes and dreams come to fruition. His desire is to help us, not hurt us, and to prepare us so that good overtakes us and not evil. God wants us to experience love, joy, peace, and a life of abundant pleasures in all areas. The truth is we are all made in the image and likeness of God. We possess His character AND creative qualities. We are fearfully and wonderfully made, we are strong and courageous, we are victorious, and we are able to overcome every obstacle that life throws at us... if we tap into the God power that lies within us.

There is absolutely nothing that God cannot do. He lives in each and every one of us, and we are made just like Him, so there is nothing that we - you and I - cannot do. Despite what others say about us or how we feel at any given time, *this is the truth about us*.

So many things happen to us in life that make us doubt who and whose we really are. These experiences cause us to disassociate with our true core, our God nature. This is one of the main reasons I wrote this book: to help others remember their true origins and put their lives - your life! - in proper perspective and context.

We must separate ourselves from the things that have happened to us. No matter what we have gone through in the past, those things do not define who we are. Just because we failed at one thing does not make us failures. Although we have lost some things, we are not losers. We may have been abused physically, mentally, emotionally, or spiritually - but that does not make us victims - we are survivors!

CHAPTER 1

CHILDHOOD, WHERE EVERYTHING BEGINS

On November 14, 1944, I was born to the union of John and Phyllis Cox and I was their sixth child. Growing up, I remember feeling free and happy as a child... but the older I became, the more self-aware I became, and I withdrew into a shell. I sadly remember losing that carefree feeling of childhood delight, and taking on the fear and insecurities of my surroundings.

Most of us have experienced some form of pain or disappointment in our lives; this is not uncommon. I can say that I have experienced more than my fair share of childhood trauma... you will learn more about that in the chapters to come. In order to progress though, I must prepare you so you have a holistic view of what happened, why it happened, and who I am because of all that occurred. To this end, I would like to share a true and accurate account of my life - my story and my testimony.

I learned some valuable lessons throughout my life. One such lesson was that I had to change the way that I thought about myself, my life, and my future if things were going to change. I could no longer view myself through the warped lens of my past. I had to embrace a new truth: what happened to me did not define me, nor did those ill-intentioned people who spoke negatively about me. The latter was harder to accept: the memories of those negative people's voices played over and over in my mind. Every time I tried to accomplish a goal that I set for myself, my mind replayed negative statements in the form of those voices to me. When I would take a step towards a goal, I heard internal voices say, "You're illiterate, you will never be anything and you will never do anything but be a housewife." I learned to fight back against those voices, to talk back and say with strength, "Oh no, I am well able! I am intelligent, strong and courageous."

I can tell you now that I have accomplished great things in spite of my insecurities, and I know that the best is yet to come! I am on my way to experiencing all of my dreams and I am happy... truly happy. But this joy in my soul only came to be by taking a serious look at my entire life - my childhood experiences, my addictive behaviors, and my progress (or lack thereof) towards my goals - and acknowledging the distinct pattern of situations and circumstances that needed to be addressed and rectified. This realization caused me to pay close attention to what was really going on in my life and make changes for the better.

The reoccurring scenes played over and over again for the better part of the first 30 years of my life. It has just been within the last 20 years that I have been able to stand on my own and be confident in who I am. Once I got away from all of the dysfunction, particularly relationships with others, I started to realize my value and ultimate self-worth. Before that point, I was simply trying to please everyone else and ended up being a doormat in the process - run over, abused, and forgotten.

To finally end this cycle, I had to identify the root causes of the patterns of abusive relationships and extended periods of depression. I had reoccurring negative thoughts of self doubt, insecurity, and worthlessness that stemmed from having low self-esteem. I felt unloved, unintelligent, and unworthy of having good things happen to me. Those negative thoughts terrorized me and caused me to self-destruct over and over again.

I finally realized that it was my responsibility to take control of the direction that my life was going in and make some serious changes. The first and most important set of changes occurred in my mind. I had to change my outlook on my life and everything that had happened and was happening to me. I had to change my perception and perspective about the way I saw myself. I started seeing myself as a person worthy of love and a good life. I started seeing myself as a victor instead of a victim. I started to see myself accomplishing the goals that I had envisioned in my mind. I really started to believe that all things were possible for me! Once I shifted my thoughts about myself, I started to see a shift in my life for the good.

In order to move forward, we sometimes have to take a look back at our past, into our childhood, as this is truly where everything begins. We learn to be what we are taught as children. We model what we see, and often times we act it out. By taking a look back into our childhood, we gain knowledge and insight as to the images and messages that have shaped our thinking, whether for good or bad. If we never address incorrect thought patterns that we sometimes learn at a young age, we will carry them over into our adulthood where they will wreak havoc.

CHAPTER 2

I AM MY MOTHER'S DAUGHTER

My mother and I never had a close relationship, and we never bonded. As a child, I was always afraid and intimidated by her. My mother was the root of a lot of pain in my life. I am not sure if my mom really liked kids. I think she had us because my dad really loved children. My mother rarely showed me love and I resented her for not being affectionate. I viewed her as selfish and self-centered, and I vowed never to be like her.

I did not care much for my mom's mothering skills. I felt she was a poor excuse for a mother. She managed the house well, but emotionally, she abandoned, neglected, and abused me both verbally and physically. When she did pay attention to me, I wished she had not because in those moments I felt like her personal slave rather than her daughter. My mom seemed to have the attitude that everyone owed her. She grew up privileged and felt that others should basically serve her and she did not need to reciprocate. My dad would try as best he could to help me when my mom would say ugly things to me or take things too far while disciplining us kids, but he did not stand a chance with her when she was heavy in her emotions, which was pretty much every day.

Without fail, my mom would just find a reason to beat on me. It seemed like she enjoyed it. I mean, if I broke a jar or tore my dress while climbing trees (I was a tomboy) she would beat me. I would wake up to beatings from her because I would suck my thumb while I was asleep. If she was not beating me, she was fussing at me, downgrading me, and making me feel as if I had no purpose in life.

My mom always seemed to point out what I was bad at, but never seemed to acknowledge what I was good at. She never took the time to find out what I could be good at. I wanted to take piano lessons, but she would not allow me to do it as a child. In her eyes, all I could do was keep the house clean. Her biggest dream for me was for me to grow up, get married and have children.

I just wish she would have taken the time to get to know me - her daughter - and to realize my skills and talents. She would have been amazed to find out that I was a budding artist - I grew up to create great sculptures, draw sketches, and paint abstract paintings. She would have been amazed to know that years later I would be a highly sought after make-up artist for major television productions, that I would own several businesses, that I would create beauty product lines, and that I would be featured as a historical civil rights leader who helped pave the way for minority business owners, particularly those who aspired to work in television, media and the film production industry.

Growing up, I had no time of relief: home was bad and so was school. I seemed to go from one bad situation to a worse one. In school, I was made to sit apart from the others as they had determined I was a "slow student". This was very hard for me because I was made to feel different than my peers from grades one through four. I was labeled as a "special needs child" and was assigned books that were just for the slow learning kids. This made it obvious to everyone that I had a different educational journey than my peers. There is a reason that I was educationally behind the rest of my peers and it was not that I was "slow." I was registered in school early, a year before I was technically eligible to enter the first grade. My mom moved some things around on the paperwork to make this happen. I never went to kindergarten and I was not prepped for first grade, but I was thrown in there at the age of five not knowing anything that five year olds know in the first grade. I had no knowledge of my ABC's, 1-2-3's, or basic kindergarten teachings that help kids adjust to an elementary classroom setting.

At home, I had no help with my school work. My mom did not help, and tried to shift the responsibility to my siblings by yelling, "Go help that girl with her school work." Well, they had no interest or time to help me and they were quick to let me know it. My siblings would call me "stupid and dumb" all the time, most notably one of my brothers. I was made to feel as dumb as bricks simply because I was a child who needed help with my school work.

I felt embarrassed because of the stigma that came along with being categorized as a child with a learning disability. The reality was I did not actually have a learning disability, nor was I illiterate as others called me; I just lacked the necessary help with my academics as other kids had available to them.

The teachers that taught us were overtaxed, as there were as many as 40 students to one teacher in our classes, and they did not have the assistance of a teacher's aide as they have now. They also did not have time to assist children like me who needed extra attention, so we just got passed along through the system. This left me and many other children at a huge educational and vocational disadvantage. I can honestly say that I never learned most of the basic things that children my age learn in school, but I graduated with my class anyway.

I knew that I was not prepared for the world, but I went on to business school. I knew in my heart that I still had what it took to succeed despite my academic shortcomings, and I had to do something to make a better life for myself. I just wanted to continue my education. I felt that if I was still being taught that I could still learn. I dedicated my time and efforts over the next several years to educational programs and professional training schools that pushed me to succeed in the areas of my passions.

Although my mom was home all day long, when we (my siblings and I) returned home from school, we would have to do all of the chores: cooking, cleaning, and catering to her every want and need. Every Wednesday was wash day. While other kids were getting ready for school, we were doing laundry. My sister, brother and I would have to get up before daybreak to wash the clothes before we went to school... while my mom was still in the bed. Laundry back then was hard work - we did not have the modern-day conveniences of automatic washing machines and dryers. Washing the clothes required us to fill double machines and tubs with water. Drying the clothes required us to hang them outside on a drying line. When it was really cold outside, the clothes would freeze by the time we hung them out.

Most times we would run late for school doing chores. My mom would get up just to tell us that she would not write an excuse letter for our tardiness because she got us up in plenty of time to complete the laundry in time. My dad would step in and tell her to "leave those kids alone so that they can get ready for school." She would concede and we would have a few minutes to prepare for school and make it there in the nick of time. The rest of the chores - the ironing, folding, and putting away of the clothes - had to be done by Saturday.

My mom shopped all the time and bought very expensive things for herself. She would buy us clothes for Christmas, Easter, back to school, and Fourth of July. These were very exciting times for me as a child. I wondered with joy, "Would we get nice things?" The answer was always, "Yes," but the quality was nowhere near the same as the clothes my mom had. I thought this was normal as a child: since my mom came from a wealthy family, I thought it was natural that she had better than we did and that she always had to have the best. My mom would walk around with minks and furs, leather gloves, and fine linens all of the time. This was just who she was. Her father purchased her first car when she was only 12 years old. Her parents ordered her clothes out of a catalog from other states. Her dad was a millionaire - literally - a successful black businessman. This was the family that she came from, a privileged family.

But my father eventually got tired and pushed back. My dad got tired of her nagging him about wanting more money, fussing at us kids all the time, and just being cruel to everyone. My mother abandoned us all for about a month after she and my father got into it - it was really bad. But I must say, while she was gone, the house ran so smoothly.

About this same time, I decided to go to business school. I was and am particularly proud of this accomplishment. My mom did not have a lot of faith in me, as she did not seem to believe that I would be successful. I pushed past that, as something inside me told me otherwise and I chose to listen to the voice within and pursue my dreams of becoming a successful business woman. Once I made that decision, I received guidance and encouragement from my older sisters, and my maternal grandmother, who always nurtured and cared for me, and stood by my side. I cannot say that my sisters' and grandmother's love filled the void created by my mother's lack of caring, but it did help. I appreciate their places in my life as loving women.

Having never experienced the natural bond of deep love that most mothers and daughters share, I have felt a void in my heart for most of my life. I missed out on experiencing a mother's love as a child, and as an adult for that matter. I have no idea what it feels like. When my mom died, I did not cry. I did not feel anything.

Lessons Not Learned At Home

My mom taught my sisters and I how to cook, clean, and be house wives; but when I left home, I was not equipped for the world that I was venturing out into. I knew nothing about managing finances, and I had a limited education with no street smarts. As kids coming from a small town, my siblings and I were often confined to the house, so I would say that we were pretty sheltered. We could only play within our own block. If mom yelled for us and we did not hear her, we were too far from the house... and we would get spanked.

I mentioned that my mom mistreated my father. She was just as unloving to him as she was to us. Sadly, in trying not to be like my mom, I overextend myself to care for undeserving men in my romantic relationships. I would give and give to them, only to have them take and take from me. They did not reciprocate my love. I see now that I dated men who were just like my mom - selfish and self-centered - trying to rewrite our relationship. It was a process to come to this realization.

Looking back, I realized that I took unnecessary crap from many men in my life, thinking that I was being kind. My "kindness" led to them walking all over me. I was frustrated by this brutal cycle and could not understand why I drew men who behaved just like my mom when I gave love just like my dad. I kept asking myself, "Why don't I draw loving and caring men like dad?"

Right before I left home, my mother told me, "Don't take a wooden nickel." Well, I knew the difference between a wooden nickel and a metal one, but I did not know what she meant. By the time I figured it out, I had taken a whole bunch of wooden nickels!

Forgiveness

I forgive my mom for the way she raised me. I feel that she did not know how to be a good mother even though she herself had a great mom. I had to forgive my mom for the way she was, because if it was not for her I would not be the person I am today.

17

CHAPTER 3

HURT & PAIN, MY FIRST MEMORIES

One should never underestimate the effects that our childhood experiences have on our mental and emotional development, and ultimately our ability to operate effectively in life. Our early years are the most impressionable ones; and often times we gather messages from our caregivers about who we are, what we are capable of, and how we should relate to the world. If those messages were not grounded in love as evidenced by positive affirmations, guidance, support, and encouragement, then we usually will not be equipped to face life with a proper perspective.

As a child, it was not unusual for me to hear my loved ones say openly that I was retarded and that I would not be able to learn or succeed like others. I eventually left my parents' home to go and live on my own, but these messages stuck with me throughout my life and haunted me daily on a subconscious level. I did not always understand why I felt insecure, incompetent, shy, or just not good enough. Now I understand that those messages spoken into my ears long ago had taken root and created mental blocks in my mind. These mental blocks affected me deeply, but did not prevent me from being able to envision positive things for myself.

People around me seemed to believe the things that my mother said about me. For example, while living in New York after leaving my parent's home at the age 19, I stayed with my sister who had left home one year earlier (also at the age of 19). When I would go out with my sister looking for employment, my sister would always take me to places that were hiring for minimum wage and mediocre skills. I was never exposed to positions that would allow me to grow and develop my natural abilities or showcase my God-given good looks.

My sister took me to a factory for my first job. I am not saying that there is anything wrong with working in a factory, but it just was not for me. I felt that she really did not know what I was truly capable of. People approached me all the time for modeling opportunities as I was slender, attractive and had a certain look that the fashion world was looking for... but being a young girl from a small town in the South, I was very intimidated, shy, and afraid to venture out and pursue modeling opportunities on my own.

I remember being approached on 42nd street in Times Square by a middle aged man who gave me his business card and asked me to call and make an appointment to come into his office and model for him. He wanted me to wear my hair in a "natural" hairstyle (at that time, I did not know what he meant by "natural" because I had never seen anyone with that style before). Once I found out, I could not imagine myself in public with my hair in a natural state, so I did not follow up on that opportunity.

New York was and still is the hub for various jobs in the fashion and beauty industry. My sister knew this and although she was not as tall and slender as me, she was obtaining modeling opportunities for herself. I did not understand why she did not push me more in that direction as she had the connections to assist me to be successful in this area. This made me feel low, like I was not on her level. I really wished that my sister would have believed in me more, but thankfully I believed in myself. I only wish I had had the confidence to go out and get those modeling jobs on my own. Instead, I went back home and back under my mother's unkind thumb.

One of the greatest emotional effects of hearing negative words spoken over me early in life was the development of low self esteem. This affected everything else in my life, especially relationships - personal and professional. I seemed to attract people who reinforced the negative beliefs that others had implanted in me as a child and young adult. Relationship after relationship exhibited a pattern of abuse, negativity and utter dysfunction - just like my childhood.

CHAPTER 4

THE LOVE OF A FATHER

The worst day of my life was the day I lost my father, John Cox, to a car accident. He was the kindest, most giving soul I have ever known. He gave his life helping others. After he died, I questioned God, asking, "Why did you take the only parent who I knew loved me?"

I loved my dad so much and he loved me. He loved all of his kids and we felt it. My mom used to say that her kids gave him all the love and gave her all the trouble. And everyone loved my dad. My father was a strong human being who had compassion for others. He always put others first. He showed me a gentle side of life when I was younger; he called me his "Peach Pie."

Loving and Kind

When it was time for my dad to come home from work, although we could not tell time, we somehow knew when it was time for daddy to arrive home, and we would run down the street to meet him. I remember being overcome with joy when I would see his head pop over the hill as he walked up the street towards our house. He had his lunch bucket in his hand and we all were anxious to see who he would let carry it home that day. We would rush out of the house and run full speed ahead to go meet our daddy. As we ran up to him, he would grab one of us up in his arms while another hung on his leg and another swung from his free arm. If my daddy took two sandwiches to work, he would bring part of his lunch back for us to have.

Although my mom made me feel like I did not matter, my dad made me feel special. I recall a time when I had gotten fed up with the abuse that I endured at home from my mom and began my plan to move out and start a new life. My mom tried to stop me from moving out of the house, saying to me, "You went to New York and did not stay, so you are not going to leave this house again until you marry out." Previous to that, I had never spoken up for myself, let alone to my mom, but this time I knew I had to stand up for myself. I said to her, "I'm not going to get married to anyone at this time and I'm going to San Francisco!"

My mom was shocked that I spoke back to her and in such an assertive manner. She ran and told my dad that I was going to San Francisco. My dad, who always yielded to my mom in the running of the house and decisions regarding the children, came to my aid.

He came to me and said, "I hear that you are thinking about going to San Francisco?"

I told him, "Yes, I'm going because I must get away from her because she is driving me crazy. If I stay here, I would be in a mental institution or I would be dead from suicide."

My dad replied, "If you feel this way, then you must go."

Then he asked, if I had enough money to get to my next destination. I told him yes, but my dad knew better - he secretly put money to the side to ensure I made it to San Francisco.

My dad gave me the money and said, "You go 'head on to San Francisco, but when you get there and find out that you don't like it, remember that you always got a home to come back to."

The threat of suicide was not just me blowing off steam, I really meant it. A lot was going on at this time with me emotionally, and I was ready to check out. I had recently been left at the altar by a high school sweetheart. This experience was traumatic, and although it happened almost two years prior to my "San Francisco stand," I was still in a lot of pain. My next relationship only intensified the pain that I felt, as I entered into a courtship with someone who became my first "true love."

About a year into the relationship, I became pregnant and he made it clear to me that he did not want any kids. He persuaded me to have an abortion. At this time, abortions were not legal and he took me to an unlicensed person who performed the procedure on me. The abortion was unsuccessful and I ended up in the hospital, almost at the point of death. And although my dad could not stand this guy's guts, especially after seeing me in the hospital from this abortion procedure, I stayed with him for a while after being released from the hospital. Thankfully, I finally got enough of him, we broke up and I decided to move to San Francisco.

With all this going on, even the love I had for my dad could not outweigh my feelings of rejection, loneliness, and pain, particularly living in the hell my mother seemed to create just for me. Death seemed like a pleasant alternative.

Chivalrous

My father was always a present help for me in my time of need. My father was a quiet man, but he was very protective of his family. He showed me how real men look out for and take care of their loved ones. He also showed me that chivalry was not dead. In the winter time, he would warm up all of the cars for the ladies in the house so that we would enter into a warm, ready-to-go vehicle. These small, but big things meant so much to me, even now as an adult. I realize my dad taught me through his actions how men should treat women. They should be treated gently, kindly, lovingly, and with much consideration of their feelings and emotional needs.

My dad showed us all of those things; he took care of his family, cared for the women in it, and showed us the utmost respect as his most prized possessions. Oh, how I love and miss him. As great of a father and husband my dad was to my mom, my mom did not necessarily support him in the same way that he supported her. She often took advantage of his kindness, good heart and non-confrontational attitude. My maternal grandmother saw how my mom treated my dad and she did not like it at all. Although she got on my mom about her need to be a better wife to such a good husband, it fell on deaf ears and she never changed: she gave that man hell at times while he continued to try to give her heaven on earth by trying to please her.

My grandmother loved my dad. She did not get along very well with my mom, her own daughter, but she had a special relationship with my father. She appreciated the good in him and how wonderful he was: an excellent provider, care-taker, loving father and a sweet soul. He went out of his way to make sure that those around him were very well taken care of, often times with not much thought to his own needs. He had no problem putting himself last and even going without for others who may have been in need. He was a selfless man.

Hardworking and Loving

I remember my dad coming home on payday, and presenting my mother his entire paycheck. He did not even cash it, he would just sign it and hand it to her. He left it to my mom the responsibility to take care of all the household needs and the luxury to do whatever else she needed. My mom did not give my dad one dime out of his own check. He would find other odd jobs, like working for my aunt and grandmother, to put a little change in his pockets.

When my grandmother would call my dad to do odd jobs around the house, he would drop everything and take care of it for her. He did the same thing for my great-aunt Ducey and others who needed him. When my grandmother would pay my father, she never told my mother about it. He would come home and my mom would ask him, "What did momma give you?" He would respond, "She didn't give me nothing." She would say, "You are telling a lie," then she would call her mother and ask, "Momma, what did you give Daddy today?" (That is what my mom called my father, 'Daddy'.) My grandmother would quickly say she did not give my dad anything, which would set my mom off! My mother would call them both liars and pitch a pure fit.

It was so sad that my mom did not think that his entire paycheck was enough for her, that she actually wanted the additional monies that he made, too. Although my mom ran the house and used the money to pay the necessary bills, she spent the remainder on excessively expensive clothing, and created astonishingly large bills at the high-end department stores in Birmingham to support her need to impress others with fine clothes and such. She did not seem to care that the large bills she ran up on herself affected everyone, especially my dad who worked very hard to support us.

Always There When I Needed Him

I am so thankful for my dad. He literally saved my life during my teenage years. This one night, I had gotten so sick that I could not get back to sleep. I got up, moaning and groaning, and my mom heard me. I ended up lying out on the floor in excruciating pain. I was not sure what was going on, but I knew that I had not felt this type of pain in my stomach before. My mom tried to give me home remedies, but it would just come back up as soon as I took it. Nothing was working and the pain did not ease up. Later on, my dad arrived home from work and saw the condition that I was in. He immediately rushed me to the hospital. When we got there, they admitted me and said that if I had not gotten to the hospital when I did, my appendix would have burst and it could have been fatal. I thank God my dad came home when he did and got me the medical attention that I desperately needed.

Protector

Daddy made our house a home. We felt cared for, safe and secure knowing that he was present and would do everything in his power to protect us. Every night, my dad would go through the entire house to make sure that all of us kids were tucked in well and that all the doors were locked before he went to bed. Not only was our natural health important to him, but our spiritual health as well. I did not understand the importance of having a strong spiritual foundation then, but now I do and appreciate the seeds of God's Word that were planted in me as a child.

Spirituality was one area that my parents were unified in. They both placed high value on building a family based on the love of God. They both made sure that we attended church every week as a family. I remember as a young girl, every Sunday my parents ensured we spent quality time giving thanks to and learning the ways of God. On Sundays, we were in church basically all day long! I did not particularly like being in church all day, but as I grew older I understood why my parents insisted on us spending so much time at church, and I gained an appreciation for that time and regarded it as precious. That is where I connected to and began my relationship with God, the most important relationship that I would ever have. Without God, I know that I would not have made it through the years of personal struggles, emotional turmoil, and all of life's challenges.

Role Model

When I thought about an ideal mate, I thought about having a man like my father. My dad showed us how to live by being a good example to us. He taught us morals and values and how to be people of integrity. He was physically and emotionally present with all of his children. Although he worked long hours and spent a lot of his spare time trying to make extra money to provide for us, he was involved in the day to day issues of our lives as best he could be. My dad was an active disciplinarian, but very different from my mom. He disciplined us from a more nurturing place than she did. While her approach was yelling, belittling, and beating us; he would punish us by giving us extra chores to complete or not allowing us to do things that we enjoyed most, such as making us stay inside all day during the summer while other kids were out having fun. I am not saying that my dad was a big softy, but I can count on my hands the times that my dad physically disciplined me. I guess that just was not his preference.

I remember one time, my sister stayed out past her curfew and my mom did not let her in the house to go to sleep. It was in the middle of winter and my mom locked her out in the freezing cold. When my dad arrived home from working an 11pm to 7am shift and saw my sister lying outside on the porch in the swing, he got so upset. I am not sure if I had seen my father this angry before. He told my mother that no matter what, she better not ever leave his children outside in the cold again. On the flip side, he got my sister straight, too: he told her that she better not break curfew again and that she better get her butt in the house on time in the future as the house rules stated. I respected my dad because he was fair and just with disciplining all of the children.

Another time, I remember my sister told my dad that I had said a curse word. He got on me and told me that I better not use that type of language and that I should have respect for him and his house. I will always remember that. He whipped my butt good, too! I guess I had really pushed his buttons with that type of language.

My dad loved his grandchildren so much! When too much time had elapsed and he had not seen the grandkids, my dad would have one of us call my sister to send the kids over. They lived close by and the kids were old enough to walk over alone. He would have their favorite foods out. While we would be on the phone calling to request the kids from my sister for my dad, my mom would be in the background yelling, "Let them kids stay where they are… I ain't up for no kids today, let them chullens stay at home, I get sick of chullens." When the kids got there, we all ended up having a good time as a family and it was memorable thanks to my dad's extra efforts to bring us all together.

Humble

My mom was the one who ran the house; she would buy everything for my dad as he did not like to go out. He was very bashful and to himself. Except this one Christmas when he came out of his comfort zone and went shopping with us. It was so special and I felt like I was on top of the world having him out with us during the holiday. He also seemed like he was actually having a blast, so that just put the icing on the cake. Another time, he drove with us to Houston, Texas. This was big because my dad really did not like being out in public. The Jim Crow laws made him very uncomfortable and intimidated him to a degree. I remember a funny story about the first time we ever stayed at a hotel. We had gone out of town to attend a funeral and while at the family visitation during the evening time, my dad warned us to hurry and get back to the hotel because in his mind, if we did not get back before it got too late, the hotel staff would lock us out. We all just laughed and laughed and had to assure my dad that we could indeed return to our hotel rooms any time we pleased as there was no curfew. That memory still makes me chuckle.

Good Son

I mentioned before that my dad and grandmother had a special relationship; they were really close. It seemed like my maternal grandmother had actually birthed my dad instead of my mom. I recall an unforgettable bonding time between my dad and grandmother. It was a time that showed how deeply they cared for each other and would sacrifice their personal fears to support the other's needs. My dad took his first flight with and for my grandmother. Although my mom was with them, too, this was huge because my father was afraid to fly. Yet, he went to Gary, Indiana to my grandmother's brother's funeral. This meant so much to my grandmother, as she would not fly without him - it was both of their first airplane flights. My grandmother trusted him so much and he cared for her to the point that they both were always there for each other in real times of need.

Excellent Provider

My dad was a country boy. He loved doing things the natural way. Even though we were not supposed to have farm animals because we lived in the city, my dad kept a full garden, raised most of our food, and my mom would store up the food by canning and freezing it so we would have food year round. I used to get upset because we had home grown stuff: brown eggs straight from the chicken and certain parts of the meat like pork and beef were smoked in the smoke house. Looking back, I realize how much pride my dad had in taking care of us, making sure that we had all that we needed. He was a great provider.

Patient

My mom said several times that she did not love my dad when they got together, that she grew to love him with time. She said that her mother and father made her marry him because they knew that my dad was a great provider. I was told that my dad's mother did not want my dad to marry my mom because she was privileged and she knew that my mom would work her son to death to maintain her lifestyle.

I did not know my paternal grandparents at all. On my mom's side, I only knew my grandmother. I heard so many stories about my maternal grandfather. I heard he was a womanizer and put my grandmother, with her sweet self, through so much hurt and pain. My grandmother would often compare my mom to my paternal grandfather, calling her selfish just like her dad. My mom would respond, "I'll take that as a compliment."

My dad was so real; he was never concerned about what people thought about him. My mom, on the other hand, was always concerned about what others thought about her. She enjoyed getting compliments from people about her looks, and she spent most of our money to maintain them. My dad would give us lunch money when he could so that we could have lunch at school, but most of the time, my mother would take all of his money to use at her discretion. The money was rarely spent on us kids specifically. Mom spent most of the money on herself, dressing up to impress people. The cars that she drove were always top of the line, again because image was very important to her. In the fifties, with lots of small kids, she was driving a Cadillac, which was considered a luxury car. I am not saying that there is anything wrong with driving nice cars, but when you have nine children, I just feel that they deserve to be a financial priority.

How I miss my father! His kindness, gentleness, and love were the oasis in the desert of my early life. I appreciate the loving person he raised me to be and am forever thankful for his protection and strength.

NEW CHAPTER 5

THE WOMEN WHO DEFINED MY EARLY LIFE

My Mother...

My Skin

I do not like to say it, but my mom differentiated between her kids. She seemed to favor my siblings that were more 'fair skinned' and the boys. That left me completely out. I was not a boy and I was not light-skinned. My mom told me directly that, "Light-skinned people are prettier than dark skinned people." It made me so angry. This was during a time when lots of black people were buying skin bleach to lighten their skin to be more accepted in society. Since the whites were the ones with all of life's rights and pleasures, being white was only right. We were made to feel from our own communities and from all media messages that being black was wrong and hopeless. Hearing that I was not beautiful, capable, or white really made me question myself. It confused me as a child and confirmed that as a people, more often than not, we had many challenges with our identity. This showed me the importance of parents, more specifically minority parents, teaching their children how beautiful, important and intelligent they are. As kids, we need to hear continuously from our parents how valuable, capable and worthy we are as *black* children. We need to hear that we deserved the best of the best.

We are the originators of so much world innovation, but the enemy has stolen our recognition. The United States was built on the backs of our people, our land was stolen, and wealth reserved for the select few. The American History books do not tell us the whole truth about the value and contribution of black people in society. We must take it upon ourselves to search out the truth, find our roots, and learn about how special we really are as a people so that we can pass the truth on to the next generation. They must have things to be proud of and see people who look like them doing great things throughout history. We must tell them of their greatness, their power and their potential.

My Education

The Holy Scriptures tells us that, "My people are destroyed because they lack knowledge." Thankfully my parents did agree on this. They taught us the importance of education and told each of us that we must finish high school and if we did not go to college, we must get a job. Out of nine children, all nine finished high school, five went on to obtain college degrees and two obtained their master's degrees.

After high school, I went on to Booker T. Washington Business College in Birmingham. About this time, my mom had been gone for about a month because she and my father had gotten into a heated argument and decided to separate for a while. When my mom returned from 'running away from home', she told me she did not intend for me to go to college, she intended for me to get a job. I did not allow this to sway me. A year and a half later, I moved to New York. When that did not work out, I tried San Francisco where I attended Hills College. There, I got a certificate in Key Punch Operation in 1967. When I moved to LA, I went to LA City College and majored in Music. I took up Make-Up Artistry at Elegance, an academy for professional Make-up Artists. Contempo School of Beauty in Inglewood, California was my next stop and I received my Cosmetology License there. When I moved to Birmingham, I began a program for Computer Information Systems at Lawson State College. In both LA and San Francisco, I took literacy courses to assist me with my reading skills. I was serious about my educational and professional goals, and I was always on a mission to better myself.

Gaining educational and career training is necessary in life. We should never stop evolving and growing as people in all areas of our lives, especially in developing our skills and talents. Thankfully, today there are a lot of tools, a wealth of free knowledge, and resources on the internet to assist people like me who are literacy deficient, to read better.

I look at people who read well and have natural skills and talents, or have extensive professional training and do nothing with themselves. It annoys me to see people throw away great opportunities. It seems that lots of folks take having a good education or outstanding talent in one area or another for granted and it upsets me. You see, I struggled all through life with my learning disability, but I took on academic goals to challenge myself. I have been determined to excel in spite of this handicap. Thank God that I did it!

I became a success in the things that I set out to do in spite of not being able to read well. If I did it, you can, too. There were a few things, however, that continue to haunt me to this day. Although I took academic challenges on, fear was still a very present force working against me professionally. I felt that people would find out that I could not read well or spell, and this affected my social and professional life. My low self esteem caused me to look up at them and down at myself. It also blocked me from fully expressing who I was and articulating my true thoughts among 'the learned.' For example, I would not talk much in a crowd of professionals for fear that I would make a mistake in pronunciation or use words out of context. That kept me from being as aggressive as I could have been as a business woman. Sometimes I would let great opportunities pass me by. Although I could do the job, I was afraid that people would find out that I could not read well and let me go. Although I read much better now, I still struggle pronouncing certain words, so I continue to stretch myself in this area. I keep a positive mindset about my abilities to grow and perfect my literary skills.

I attended first grade at Robinson Elementary School in Fairfield, Alabama, the suburbs of Birmingham. I did not go to kindergarten as my mom basically threw me in school by changing some of my enrollment documents. I was only five years old and the other kids were six, which was the school's age requirement for first grade. My peers were older and had been prepped for this new educational experience by kindergarten, but I had not. I had no clue what was going on most of the time in class and felt lost and out of place.

My mom did not explain anything to me about school and I was not prepared when I got there. The elementary school environment was absolutely foreign to me. While the other students seemed to be getting along perfectly, I was terrified. I was bashful and shy. I did not like school. Every day I woke up and prepared to go to school, but would cry for one reason or another. My excuse for not wanting to go to school was anything: I could not find a pencil, I lost a shoe, I was sick… anything to get out of going.

My Grandmother

A Ram in the Bush

My mom never gave us a lunch to carry to school, and for breakfast each morning we would have the same thing: grits. One day, my teacher told me to go home and tell my mom to fix me lunch. My mom sent me to the store to get a loaf of bread so that I could make a peanut butter and jelly sandwich to take back to school. We only lived a couple of blocks from the school. Ultimately, this did not last and I was once again without lunch every day. My grandmother started sending lunch for me with my cousin, Arcola, as we were the same age, and in the same class. Arcola lived with our grandmother.

Thoughtful and Generous

Grandma would make Arcola and I clothes alike, and sometimes we would dress like twins. I knew that when I spent the night with grandma that I would eat good. She was a great cook. I knew that I would have a balanced meal there. It was a real treat.

I grew up on beans and bread, and only had meat sometimes. On Sundays, we usually had chicken. But even Sunday meals were sometimes lean. When my great uncle and his wife would come over unannounced and eat up most of the food that mom had prepared for Sunday dinner, it left us kids with scraps. Sadly, if you visited my uncle's house, he would not offer you anything! Mom would treat him like royalty; the children would have to sit and wait until they had finished eating and then we could have whatever was left. He would do the same thing at everyone's house that he went to, including my grandma's house. Since she did not have a lot of people to feed, grandma would have leftovers and everyone, the children and adults, would eat at the dinner table at the same time unlike at my parents' house.

I loved to visit my grandmother. She was strong, clean and kept her house in order. She was extremely kind to everyone.

During the holidays, we would all cram up in her house and had a great time. Her house was pretty small: she had about four rooms and we had a big family. I am not sure how we all fit inside, but we did. We would, as kids, do a play and act it out for the rest of the family, which were usually my mother, her sisters, and all of their children.

My Grandma saved boxes from product purchases through the year to use to wrap our Christmas gifts in. She would save all kinds of product boxes: grit boxes, washing powder boxes, oatmeal and starch boxes. When we would un-wrap our gifts, it was so exciting to see who had what type of box. We would make fun of each other's boxes jokingly saying, "Oh, you have a box of cereal," or "You have a box of starch." Those were some good times.

The gifts were nice: lotion, socks, or other personal products. In addition to the personal care products, my grandmother's baked - cakes and pies were her specialty. It made us feel so good that she thought that much about all of the people in her life to take the time to get us all something and wrap it from her heart. She not only gave all of the grandchildren gifts, but she also prepared gifts for her neighbors, too. I am still not sure how she did it all with her limited resources, but she did. Thinking back to those days brings joy to my heart, as the love and attention meant so much. We had the best times at my grandmother's house.

My Little Sister

Another source of joy in my life was and is my sister. Phillis is the younger sister right after me, and she and I are very much alike. Growing up, we looked alike, so people thought we were twins. Sometimes her classmates would see me at a distance out and about in the community, and call out her name to say 'hi'; the same thing would happen to her with my classmates. We would kindly play it off and speak to them all and just notify each other of who we ran into that day.

Our similarities also led to some comedic moments. When I was in college at Booker T. Washington, older guys would try to talk to Phillis, who was still in high school thinking she was me. It was so funny to see them falling all over themselves trying to get her attention. She did not help matters - she used my age and identity to make the guys think that she was older than she was, and it worked, too.

Loving and Loyal

My sister was and is very sensitive. You can say "boo" and make her cry. But she is also a kind soul and unfortunately, people take advantage of her kind spirit. Throughout her life, she has always freely given her time, talent, and love, and never demanded anything in return. She is also very low key and "goes with the flow".

My sister is a loyal person: she was at one job for 18 years and the next job for about 16 years. In addition to being a dedicated worker, she assisted financially with the raising of her three grandchildren as her son - their father - was strung out on drugs for over twenty years. My sister's nurturing and generous spirit was not just limited to her son and grandchildren - it also thankfully included me. I remember going home for visits through the years and being showered with so many gifts that I did not have enough room to receive them - literally! I had to tell her to stop giving me clothes and shoes, as I could open up a shoe store with all of the shoes that she had given me. My sister seemed to always look beyond her own needs to provide for the needs of others. That is what makes her so very special; she was and is so much like my dad.

Tenacious

I love my sister's determination. She is a fighter, a true warrior! She has overcome breast cancer, rectal cancer and a brain aneurism. She even overcame a terrible fall when she was trying to get some things out of the attic for my brother's birthday party. Her ankle was crushed and she had pins placed in it to hold her ankle to her leg. She is an over-comer, a survivor and very much loved. When I look at her life and how she has kept moving in faith with a positive attitude in spite of adversity, I am inspired. The fact that she reminds me so much of myself and my dad creates in me a strong sense of connection. I feel my father lives on in us, as we both carry beautiful characteristics learned from him.

The Women of the Church

Ms. Moore was one of the mothers of our church. She used to love when I sang *I Shall Not Be Moved*. She was such a sweet, pleasant person and had such a gentle spirit. Ms. Moore always had a smile on her face. I still remember her smile. It made me feel significant and appreciated at a time when all around me was going wrong.

Ms. Moore's daughter, Ms. Josie Carson, was over the youth at our church. She told me years ago that I needed to write a book about my life. I was only 18 at the time, and had just gotten out of jail from a march related to the Civil Rights Movement with Dr. Martin Luther King, Jr. Ms. Carson told me that my life was significant. She was a source of strength, and told me - and the other youth - how important we were in Christ.

Ms. Josie's words were seeds of encouragement. Although it took me many years to do it, I wrote this book based on the seeds planted long ago by Ms. Josie. Her belief in me and the gifts that she saw within me, even when I did not see them, were balms to my soul. People like her are priceless blessings to us on our journey to become our best selves. They speak life into our ears that ignite inner dreams and visions.

Be thankful for the people who God places in your life, people who motivate you to do more, to be more, to live to your fullest potential. You may not think words of affirmation such as "You are great," "There is greatness within you," and "You should write a book, write a song, or start your own business" mean anything, but they mean everything. They open up your mind to new possibilities that you might otherwise not consider.. They push you to look past life's limitations and to tap into the power of your potential, which is limitless.

Surround yourself with people who understand the power of words and speak life over you and your dreams. You may not see immediate results, but trust me, you will see results. As you read this book, this is a testimony of the power of positive word seeds being planted in my mind as a teenager. You do not have to take as long to move on divine inspiration as I did, but better late than never, right?

CHAPTER 6

WHY ME?

Around the age of ten I was molested. The abuse continued for over a year. The man who violated me was a well respected member of the community with children of his own. I did not tell my mother because I did not feel close enough to her to talk about anything. I did not dare tell my father because he would have killed the man and that would have left me fatherless, without the only person who showed me love at home. As a result, I suffered in silence. I kept the nasty secret to myself for years, and this deeply affected me on many levels. If I had not been made to feel worthless enough by siblings, my peers, and my mother it took a trusted male figure in my life to carve the message in my soul that, "I was worthless, damaged goods and a target for abuse." This is the way that I felt each time this person would climb on top of me, fondle my young body, then relieve himself. I was only 10 years old for heaven's sake!

Emotionally I was a wreck. I was a baby girl trying to figure out, why me? Was I the only one? Should I or could I tell anyone? If I told someone, would anyone believe me? Was this my fault? After all, we were taught religiously that you do as adults tell you. I was following the instructions of an adult, but somehow this just did not seem right to me. Eventually, I grew to know that it was not right, but I still did not know what to do about it. I could not for the life of me understand why this sexual violation was happening to me.

This was not my only experience of molestation at the hands of an older, respected man in the community. Back in those days, this type of disgusting sexual behavior was ignored - the community turned a blind eye to it and did not talk about it. In my mind, this is tacit acceptance and this flagrant disregard to child safety damaged me. Around the same time I was being violated by my family's friend, another neighborhood man took advantage of my vulnerable child state.

My mother would often times send us to the store in the late evenings. There were no street lights, just one light down the hill near the end of the block by the store, so it would be dark as we walked. My mom would be out of cigarettes or things that my dad needed for lunch, so we would have to run to the store before it closed. The old man would stand out on the sidewalk by the telegram post, taking advantage of the shadows. I could not see him until I got close to him. He would hiss at me and tell me to come to him. Out of obedience, I would go - this was what we were taught, to respect and obey our elders. He would put his hands all over me, mostly touching my behind. After he would let me go, I felt dirty, ugly, worthless and so nasty that no amount of water could clean me.

Parents, please teach your children that if someone touches them in an inappropriate manner, that they should tell you! Also, ask your children from time to time if anyone has touched them in a manner that made them feel uncomfortable. I wish I could say we can trust everyone who comes around our children, but we cannot. We cannot even trust some of our family members. We have to be very careful who we allow around our children. There are so many stories from people I know who were raped and abused for years by "trusted and respected" people in their families and communities. One male friend of mine was molested for years at the hands of a close family friend. Another was raped and abused by his Catholic Priest. It is our responsibility to watch out for our children and make sure that we do all we can to protect them and keep them from evil people.

I often wondered why so many hard things happened to me. I could not understand why I had to endure such suffering and strife. I now realize that my life experiences were not just for my own learning and development, but also to prepare me to help others who are going through difficulties. The trials I have faced and overcome have made me a stronger and better person who did not succumb to, but overcame my situations through prayer.

Life is about the storms we go through and how we weather them. Because we are either going into a storm or coming out of one, these storms are in our lives to teach us about our faith and our connection to the Higher Power. It took me many years to learn this very valuable lesson. As I matured in my spiritual life, I began to understand my connection with God. Now that I understand who I am in God, I have come to a place where I fully accept who I am and also accept who others are as well. I have learned to love myself. I no longer accept mistreatment from others or allow abuse from anyone. I completely disconnected myself from toxic and negative people and this has made all of the difference. This is not to say that I no longer get tested by others in these areas, but I now know how to deal with people who are mean, hurtful, abusive, users and just disrespectful evil-doers. I have come to understand for myself that the saying, "hurt people, hurt people" is a reality. It is unrealistic to expect to receive love from a person who does not love him- or herself because that person does not know what love is. Every person is a pipeline through which either love or hate flows. If you do not have love within, you cannot give it out. This is just a fact.

No matter how "good of a person" you are, you cannot change other people. What you *can* do is do good to others; pray for those who use, abuse, and mistreat you; and forgive them and move on. This is a necessary part of your spiritual growth, development and maturity. It is also necessary to gain the wisdom necessary to be grateful for the circumstances that allowed that wisdom to be. I am now actually thankful for the painful situations that happened to me and the growth that took place within because they have made me the person I am today. The woman I am today sees negative characteristics in others quickly, and acknowledges those "red flags" early on in a relationship. It allows me to swiftly release people from my circle who are not positive. I am able to love and minister grace to those people, but I do not allow them to mistreat me. I also speak up for myself, something I rarely did before, and I feel no guilt when I completely remove myself from negative people.

I remember a word from Pastor William (Bill) Hornaday, who I respect very much: "If you are around people who are constantly negative, putting you down, making you feel low, even if it's your mother, you better run from them like they have a plague!" Those words stuck with me and are now words that I truly live by. I honestly feel that it is better to be alone than to be around people who are not positive, operating in integrity, Godly, spiritually-minded, and on the same path as me. I learned to surround myself with people who can help me stretch, make me think, help me grow into a better person so that I may fulfill my purpose in life.

Prayer has been a major tool that has helped me to overcome obstacles in life. I am a witness that prayer works. I learned that when you pray to God (your higher power), relax, and continue to believe and work in faith, God then begins to work through and for you. You must pray, release it - whatever "it" is - completely to God, and move on in a spirit of gladness and expectation. Then God will show up and show out on your behalf. You will know that God is working behind the scenes when you have supernatural peace deep down inside.

I remember a time when God stepped in for me and answered my prayers immediately in a supernatural way. My friend Mel and I had just returned from Jamaica, and had a long layover in New York. We were invited to stay with friends - Harold and his mate George. Coincidentally, Harold was flying to Tel Aviv the next morning. Since our flights departed about the same time, he suggested we all share a cab to the airport. As we were working out the details, I got up to look for my purse and there was no purse. As I went to locate my flight itinerary, I realized that my purse was nowhere to be found. To our horror, I realized I had left my purse in the cab that had brought me to his home! All of my personal information, credit cards and money were in my purse! The itinerary for our trip was in there, too. Needless to say that this was a nightmare and everyone was scurrying looking for ways to locate my purse and the cab company that we used.

I retreated like Jesus to a place of prayer and meditation on God's Word during this time of frustration and desperate need. I prayed, relaxed, released, and started to meditate on how great my trip was going to be; I did not think about anything else. Even though at the time, I was not sure of *how* it would actually all work out, I just knew that it would. This is an example of how powerful the mind truly is. Whatever you envision, believe, and receive as done for you in your heart, you will really have it! By faith, I saw a happy ending to this story, a beautiful fun trip and was not worried about how it would happen. I left that to God. I had real peace about the situation, and guess what? God came through for us right on time and the trip was even more amazing than I had envisioned.

About an hour and a half after I went into prayer, the cab driver pulled up to Harold's house and knocked on the door. He had actually located me! Two other people had gotten into the cab after us and the last one informed the driver of the purse that was left in his cab. He said that he felt a sense of urgency to get my purse to me after he checked my driver's license and discovered that we had the same birthday: month, day, and year!

The really miraculous part is how he came to remember where he dropped us off, because of course the address on my license was not where we were staying in New York. When the cab driver picked us up from the airport, we gave him the address, and he and Mel went back and forth about the direction the driver was going because Mel thought the driver was cheating us by taking us the long way. The address stuck in the driver's head because he had to explain to Mel multiple times that although it would normally be quicker to go through Central Park, there was construction that way so we needed to take the longer route. That was God's way of letting the driver know how to find me. It was definitely a divine moment where I saw God answer my prayer. The peace that I felt before the cab even arrived is just a testament to my inner knowledge that God had heard me, and was working on my behalf all of the time. I never doubted that things would work out right in the end and they did.

Previous to that experience, I had never experienced that kind of peace. I had no worries, no doubt, or anxiety. I meditated and actually felt the experience of the plane taking off, us leaving on time as scheduled and enjoying a wonderful trip. And it all happened just like that.

You can have the same peace in your life. When mishaps, obstacles, or challenges that are out of your control happen, I suggest that you retreat to a place of prayer and let the peace of God, which surpasses all understanding, guard your heart from worry and anxiety about things not working out for you. Trust that *all* things are working for your good and believe that God always has your best interests at heart. Rest in His promises to take care of His children and wait patiently for Him to do what you cannot on your own. It is best said by this mantra: "Let go and let God."

Let God handle the details. Have faith and trust in His love for you as a good father. He is the God of the supernatural. I have learned that the key to a successful and peaceful happy life is to build your faith in God. Faith opens the door to everlasting peace. You will never find peace in obtaining material things. They come and go. The type of peace that I am talking about *only* comes through having a relationship with God and having faith and confidence in His ability to care for you as His child. The scriptures tell us that faith comes by hearing the Word of God. So, to grow in your faith, you must hear on a consistent basis the Word of God. With the internet and so many online applications, there is no reason for anyone not to be able to learn and hear God's Word. By hearing His Word which is life to our Spirit, we are empowered to believe and see the impossible become possible for us. It all happens through hearing, learning and understanding God's Word for yourself. Hebrews 11:6 teaches us "…without faith it is impossible to please God. He is a rewarder of those who diligently seek Him." It's so comforting to know that God actually rewards our faith!

CHAPTER 7

THE WEDDING THAT NEVER HAPPENED

There was a time when my life seemed to be a constant series of disappointments. The one that seems to pop out at me the most is my wedding that never happened.

I was so excited about the wedding and had been busy planning our nuptials like any giddy bride-to-be. I had selected the venue, our attire, and sent out the invitations to all of our family and friends. After growing up in a household feeling out of place, isolated, and neglected, I would finally belong to someone! I would be accepted and loved unconditionally by *my* man. My man was going to rescue me from the prison of my parent's home and I could not have been more elated about being set free!

My former fiancé was in the Navy, and one of the most exciting aspects of being a military spouse was that I would be moving with him to see and travel the world. I saw this as an opportunity to get away from my small town and the negative voices of limitation. I was excited to be a wife and I could not wait to start my new life in a place where no one knew me. It was a new beginning. I was so excited and I was happy that I was getting a "new lease" on life.

Life was perfect and I was walking on cloud nine: I was young and in love with my high school sweetheart, and we were engaged to be married. I thought that I had finally found "love" and my life would now begin to look up. I would no longer be alone. I was so excited to show my family that I could, in fact, be a successful wife and mother. The family would see that I had found my life partner and we would live happily ever after and ride away into the sunset!

My dream came to a screeching halt when my fiancé abruptly called off our wedding four weeks before our wedding date. I was devastated. I could not possibly have gotten this close to getting married only to be abandoned. I really thought that I was having a bad dream. I cannot put into words the effects of literally being left at the altar had on me, but I can say that the spectrum of emotions that I experienced almost took me out. I was hurt, embarrassed, and ultimately disappointed that my dream of having a love of my own had evaded me. I could only imagine what others were thinking and how they pitied me. After all, all I ever heard from those closest to me was that I was not smart enough, good enough, or pretty enough for anything good to come my way. When my fiancé jilted me, it was like the universe was playing a sick joke on me and mockingly saying, "Yes, your dreams can come true! You have found your ideal mate! He'll love you forever! You too will be happy! Yeah, right! Instead of expecting long lasting love, you should just expect constant disappointments, especially in the area of your romantic relationships. This whole marriage thing was just a joke! HA HA HA!" Well, a joke (on me) is definitely what it turned out to be. My ex-fiancé married someone else months later, and they had a child together shortly thereafter.

I was crushed; crushed to the point that I planned to kill myself. I had gone to the pharmacy where I used to work and gotten pills. I had already written a letter to my family and had left it in my room. I stopped by my girlfriend's house to give my final goodbyes and she ended up calling my family immediately after I left her house. Her calling my family to inform them of the suicide plan was actually how they found out that the wedding was cancelled. My family took the medication from me; they contacted a lawyer to try and recoup some of the money that was spent on the wedding to no avail; they encouraged me not to be dismayed or give up on my hopes of having a good guy. They were very supportive.

It took me some time to get beyond this low point in my life. I mean, he was my first love. I was young, in my early twenties and felt like I would never ever experience that type of love again. After all, what girl does not want to marry her first love?

The hardest part of advancing beyond the ordeal was getting over the shock and the utter embarrassment of it all. I found myself in a deep depression crying a lot. I was humiliated. All I could think was, "Why me?" I had lost so much money in the planning of this grand event. Facing everyone after sending out the notices to cancel the wedding was hard. Thankfully, my loved ones felt my pain and no one rubbed it in or made me feel worse about what happened.

As painful as it was, calling off my wedding after being so close to the actual event date ended up being one of the best things that ever happened to me. Looking back, I can honestly say that I was too young, immature, and sheltered to handle the responsibilities that would have come along with being someone's wife. I was naïve about life and had no clue about how to love another person effectively. I had experienced quite a bit of childhood trauma that negatively affected me. I had low self esteem, had not seen adequate examples of healthy relationships, and was completely unprepared for marriage because I did not know what it would involve. I just wanted to be out of my parent's home by any means necessary.

This cancelled wedding disappointment could have left a life scar in my emotions and blocked me from seeing a brighter future, one full of hope, love and even marriage. Since this was not the first time that I had been let down by love, I began to develop a negative thought pattern about my life in general. I began to think that nothing good would ever happen to me, that I would always experience failure in relationships, that I should not expect to be loved. I basically felt that my life would forever be a story of gloom and doom.

Thank God, that was not the end of it! A scripture that helped me to change the course of my life by changing the course of my thinking was Proverbs 23:7. It says, "As a man thinks in his heart, so is he." This is a very profound scripture. In short it says that whatever you think is what you become. Despite the negative events that had occurred in my life, I had to choose to change how I perceived my situation and how I thought about myself in relation to what had happened to me in the past. I had to learn to separate myself from the things that had happened in my life. Despite how I often felt, I was not my past and I was not a victim, a rejected one, or a failure. I was a survivor, an over-comer, a victor! By changing the way I thought, I was able to embrace a whole new vision of myself - one who is wiser, stronger and now using all of the things that the enemy meant to harm me as fuel to bless others through my testimony.

CHAPTER 8

RELATIONSHIP BLUES

I experienced a lot of relationship drama. I do not regret any of it because I learned valuable lessons from each person that I connected with. However, I cannot count the number of times that I have had to restart my life after a dramatic episode with guys. This just seemed to be a continuous cycle in my personal life. My romantic relationships usually involved me being used and abused by men. I wish I had learned to love myself early in life - then I would not have wasted so much time with people who did not deserve me. This is a major wisdom nugget for everyone reading this book. Time is something that you can never get back so be mindful of how and with whom you spend your time.

I remember my first romantic let down. I was in the tenth grade and Keith, an upper-classman and "big time" senior was very popular. The ladies loved him - self included. A month before the prom he asked me to be his date. I was very proud to be asked by him, and of course I said yes! I was so excited and I planned every detail - what I would wear, how I would walk, my hair, the works. I did not think about much else from that point forward. But guess what? He called me the day before the prom and told me that he could not take me. He ended up taking another girl. I was devastated, embarrassed, and felt so rejected. Thankfully, my friend Harold came to my rescue and took me to the prom. I ended up having a good time, but there was still a stain of rejection and abandonment that was hard to get over.

Later on, Keith and I reconnected and became friends again. He went off to college and I was still in high school. He went to Tuskegee and after a year his parents could not afford for him to stay. Before he could enroll into another college, he was drafted into the Army, but did not want to go so instead went into the Marines. They sent him through basic training, and while there Keith wrote me a letter saying he was going to surprise me with a visit after his training was over. On his way home, his ship was turned around and sent to Vietnam. Tragically, he was killed in Vietnam. Keith died from a gunshot wound to his leg that turned into gangrene from being left unattended. This was extremely devastating for me because this was the first time that I had experienced losing someone that close to me. It was really hard to get through, but I took it day by day and learned to go on with life. I was grateful he and I reconnected and made our peace. I realized that the world keeps moving and life goes on and so we have to keep going on, too. Nothing stops.

My next love connection was Marcus. I met Marcus after I moved back to Birmingham from New York. One morning while I was at the bus stop he offered me a ride to work. My friend and I began riding with him every morning and eventually we became a couple. Marcus even set up my girlfriend with a friend of his and we would double date sometimes. Things were really great in the beginning:

we went out every Saturday night to the same club where the infamous Clarence Carter was performing. This was a very exciting time for me. I was not accustomed to hanging out and going to the clubs and such, as I was barely legal. The clubs did not really check identification at that time and Marcus was considerably older than I, so people did not give it a second thought. Marcus often showed me a part of life that I had never experienced, mostly nightlife. This was one of the main reasons one of my brothers did not like him. Of course I did not care about my brother's opinion at that time. I was young, head in the clouds and living for me. I did not pay any attention to any of my family members who tried to offer me advice about this relationship. I even ended up having a falling out with my mom, which left us not communicating for over a year because of Marcus.

Marcus ended up being one of the most selfish people who I have ever met. It was either his way or the highway. He was a person of repetition and a true demonstration of a creature of habit. He did the same thing every day, the exact same way, and went to the exact same places every weekend. He was predictable and did not want to veer off to do anything different. At first, this was fun because it was new for me, but it soon became boring.

After I left Birmingham for San Francisco, a year later Marcus moved to LA. He called me and invited me to move down there with him. I had a great job, was doing very well, and was stable and secure. I uprooted myself and decided to move there with him. When I got to LA, he put me up in a hotel for a week and I had not visited his place once. I started to ask questions about why I had not been by his apartment yet, and he told me that we were on a honeymoon. Wow, I still cannot believe that I bought that one! Then later he confessed about a young lady that he had staying at his place that he was "helping out." He said that she would be leaving soon and asked me to be patient as he worked out that situation. The lady who he was "helping out" ended up being his girlfriend that he had brought with him from Alabama. He told me not to tell her anything about us. It was crazy. Shortly after, I headed back to San Francisco.

When I moved back to San Francisco, I got a job with a cosmetics company that allowed me to travel all over the country. I loved to travel, as it helped me to put my failed relationship behind me. After a year, I was transferred to Miami. It was amazing and I loved it: the people, the culture, and the weather were just what I needed. Unfortunately, I only stayed for a year, but oh what a year!

While in Miami, I hung out with Blanch Calloway, Cab Calloway's sister, who was the president of the company I worked for. We had some grand times! I also hung out with Dorothy Guy, whose husband used to play in Duke Ellington's band. Mr. Ellington invited us to come see him direct the Miami Symphony, and we had front row seats. He invited us to meet him backstage after the show in his dressing room. He was just lounging on his futon when we came in and he was extremely happy to see his friends Blanch and Dorothy. I told him how much we enjoyed the show, I shook his hand and we chatted casually. He was really kind and I felt so honored to meet such a legend. Times like these were plentiful while I was in Miami, but I had a calling in my spirit to do more and see more! So I moved back to San Francisco for a time. Looking back, I realize it was a mistake because it was too close to Marcus... and back I went to him, once again placing myself in a situation where I would be mistreated and abused.

About a year or so after moving back to San Francisco, and then L.A., I found that Marcus was back to his old tricks: he had another girl from Birmingham staying with him. This time, I did not keep it a secret. I told the young lady about my relationship with him *and* about the first young lady who had lived with him in secret. Marcus got so upset that he jumped on me and hit me several times. Thankfully, the young lady intervened saying that if he hit me again he would have to get to me through her. She was a bit bigger than me and looked like she could give him a run for his money, so he backed off. I gathered up some things and went to stay with my girlfriend for a while. The other young lady had obviously had enough, and high tailed it back to Birmingham. How I wish I had put my foot down, too...

Shortly after this episode, I found a job at a little boutique. I ran it for over two years, and did a very fine job. The owner, a nice Jewish man named Bob, offered to sell it to me. During this time, I had reconciled with Marcus, and once I reopened the boutique as the new owner, Marcus quit his job. Bob was an Angel in disguise - he saved me from being swindled. When it was time for me to sign the sales contract, I found out that Marcus had tried to buy the boutique right from under me! Bob made sure that did not happen when he said, "Veronica, come here - I'm not selling this store to Marcus, I'm selling it to you."

I owned the store, but did not see any of the profits. Marcus took care of all of the bank transactions, and he was in control of all the money. I ran the store for over five years and never saw a dime. Marcus did all the shopping for the store, even though it was a women's shop. Previous to his involvement, I had done all the shopping, but now Marcus insisted on doing it. It was his way of maintaining control.

My time with Marcus was rocky to say the least. Not only was he a liar, cheater, and womanizer, he also compromised my physical safety and wellbeing. When I spoke earlier about the man whose guts my dad hated, Marcus was that man. During my relationship with Marcus, I became pregnant. He did not want a baby and he persuaded me to have an abortion. Abortion was not legal back then, and many of the places that performed them were unsanitary. Non-sterile instruments were used during my procedure. I got a horrible infection that really messed me up and landed me in the hospital. I almost died from this ordeal, but it was a necessary one as it brought me to this realization: Marcus' purpose in my life was to show me the type of man I did *not* want, and that if I met a man who demonstrated similar characteristics in the future, I should run fast.

No matter how bad a situation is, there is a lesson that can be learned from it. Boy did I learn valuable lessons from Marcus. He played me for a fool. Took all of my money and had women all around me right in front of my face. I ran the store for over five years and never saw a paycheck. He took the money and squandered it at the race track (he was a gambler).

The boutique was doing well, so well that when an opportunity to purchase the shoe store across the street came available, I was able to do so. Marcus was supposed to run the shoe store and I was to run the boutique, but that never happened. He hired a senior citizen to run the shoe store while he was at the racetrack or in the streets doing whatever. Our employee would get off at 4pm and Marcus would return shortly before that to relieve her, so he was only there a couple of hours. Marcus then had the idea to consolidate the stores. The boutique made more money than the shoe store and it was in a better location. However, Marcus decided to move my boutique over to the shoe store location because the rent was cheaper.

We worked together in the consolidated location for a while and things were going okay... until I turned thirty. On my thirtieth birthday, I asked Marcus what his intentions were toward me. Were we going to remain in a non-committed relationship or was he planning to marry me? He nonchalantly responded that, "No one would force me to marry and that I'll do it when I'm ready."

When I heard the word "force", it was like someone had gut punched me. I felt dirty and low down, and it really pierced my heart and angered me. I regretted that I had not asked him this question long ago. I had wasted so many years with him, years that I could never get back. I met Marcus when I was 20 years old and I did not walk away from him until I was 30. The first five years of our relationship were on-and-off, as I would leave and come back, leave and come back. It was not until he used the word "forced" that the light bulb came on and I realized how much time I had wasted with this guy. That is when I left him.

Whenever I would disagree with Marcus, he would tell me to "get out" knowing that I did not have the means to support myself. Sometimes I would leave and go over to my girlfriend Ruth's house. Marcus would eventually come get me, moving my stuff back and we would make up. Ruth was a Japanese coworker of mine at the Fireman Fund Insurance Company, my first job in San Francisco. We were roommates for a couple of years and became really good friends. We moved to LA together: she moved in with her sister and I moved in with Marcus. We are still friends today and keep in touch. She was always there for me when Marcus would kick me out.

This time when I left, I did not care about my financial distress; I knew in my heart that God would take care of me and that I was going to be all right. I told Marcus he could have the businesses, the apartment, and all of our beautiful furniture. I went out and got a job at the local supermarket so I could get my own place. I learned from him that you need to walk away from a situation that is not going anywhere, cut your losses and just go on while you still have your mind.

As fate would have it, as soon as I left Marcus, his life fell apart. He lost everything: the businesses and the apartment. He put all the furniture in storage and moved to the slums. Everyone makes choices for themselves, and that was his.

After I had saved enough money, I got my own apartment. After a few months, I could finally enjoy the freedom that came with this small, yet hard won, battle for independence. I felt good and it was nice to have peace and personal space after leaving the drama that came with Marcus. This was a new chapter in my life and I was excited about this new beginning.

I met my next partner, Tom, while working at the supermarket. He seemed like a good person, and an ideal man I would have liked to marry. He was kind, gentle and caring; everything Marcus was not. We started dating and over the next five months or so it got pretty steady. I would visit his place and he would visit mine. He would cook for me and offer to bring it to my home so that I would have dinner after I got off work. Since he did this often, I did not think a thing about giving him the key to my apartment when one day he asked for it. It would allow him to bring food over more easily without bothering me to let him in.

One day, I got home to find Tom and all of his stuff in my apartment. I was shocked to say the least and asked him what was going on. He said that we had talked about how much each of us was spending on rent. This was true, we had talked about it in general, but there was never a conversation about him moving in with me. When I conveyed this to him, he replied by telling me that he had given up his apartment to move in with me, so what did I want him to do? I was hot because I had just gotten out of that crazy situation with Marcus and was not ready for anyone to move in with me. He told me how he did not have anywhere to go, having given up his place to stay with me, so I felt it only right to give this cohabitation with him a try.

Tom was very different from Marcus. He actually made me appreciate the small things, not just the big things that come along with having a good man. He would cook, clean, shop and take care of our household needs. We worked together. For example, if I cooked, he would wash dishes, and vice versa. Marcus would never do any of that stuff. I started to like having Tom around the apartment as my mate.

Tom was almost a perfect potential husband, except for his tendency to lie from time to time and his jealousy. He was a generous man - a great guy. He was a good lover. He was so exciting, spontaneous and adventurous; he showed me a lot of the world that I would have never seen. Sometimes we would wake up in the morning and he would say, "Where do you want to go today?" Or "What do you want to do today?" We would get up and do some of the most romantic things. It was normal for us to just get up and drive five hours to the mountains, hike through the forest, or ride bikes on a nature trail. To end a beautiful escapade, we would drive out to the ocean and watch the sun set. I never knew what to expect with Tom, but I always knew that it would be fun and fresh. I loved that about him.

Tom was also big on holidays. No matter if it was Christmas, Thanksgiving, my birthday, or Mother's Day (even though I was not a mother), it seemed like I was always being showered with gifts from Tom. Marcus on the other hand did not believe in any holidays, or so he claimed. I think he did not want to spend money on anyone but himself. But with Tom, it always felt like Christmas. He was about fifteen years older than I, and had kids almost my age. We all got along and spent lots of time together doing family outings which was a breath of fresh air for me. It was beautiful, our family time.

Tom and I did so much together; I wish I could re-live some of it. We traveled to several countries. My relationship with Tom helped me to overcome my grief when I lost my father. After my dad's funeral, Tom and I drove across country for two weeks. We took a road trip like no other: we started in Atlanta, then went to Philadelphia, hit Pittsburg (Tom's hometown), made a stop in the Maryland area to visit his daughter and tour the major historic sites in the DC area. We continued on to Canada, Niagara Falls, the Grand Canyon, Aspen Colorado, and many other places. Every Easter we would go to Yosemite National Park, and since we lived in Los Angeles, we visited a lot of the National Parks in California.

We lived together for five years, but Tom never put to rest his insecurities. And they were serious insecurities. He was a very jealous man and that jealousy was an illness. Like my mother would always say, "He's like a cow that puts out a good bucket of milk, then turns around and kicks it over." He would do good things, but then he would turn around and mess it up by being jealous. We went to all these places and had such a nice time, but he made me miserable because I would always end up upset when he would accuse me of being with somebody or looking at somebody. We could be in the car driving and I am just riding, then all of a sudden he would start puffing real loud and I knew that he was getting very upset. So I would ask him, "What's wrong with you?"

He would say, "I see you looking at that man."

And I'd respond, "We're in the car and the car is moving?!?! What man? Turn around and go back so I can see him too since he got your attention." (That was my way of saying that whoever he saw must have been fine, and I wanted to see him, too, since I really did not see anyone.) This happened all the time.

One day, he came home from work and asked, "Who's been here today? I found this red piece of hair in the bathroom." Well, the lady downstairs had red hair, and either one of us could have brought the hair in on our shoes or something. It was always silly stuff like that.

45

Tom did such beautiful things, and then messed them up with his jealousy. I recall a time that really got me fed up with him. It was during a really difficult time for me and my family. My father had just gotten killed in a car accident and we were in the process of making funeral arrangements for him. Instead of Tom being supportive and concerned about our grieving, he wanted to go sightseeing and got upset that I was not trying to show him around. That was so selfish and inconsiderate, and really showed me his true colors. I got so upset with him that I told him he could go back to California and get all of his stuff out of my place. I said that I did not want to see him when I got back there. Tom apologized, so we made up, and ended up staying together after this blow up. He smoothed things over as we traveled across the country together as I mentioned earlier. It was very therapeutic for me after losing my father so tragically.

When we returned to Los Angeles, things were okay for a while, but Tom's jealousy just continued to get worse. I started to feel miserable most of the time because of the ups and downs that we constantly went through. I recall a turning point in our relationship. We went to visit a girlfriend of mine who had recently escaped a very abusive relationship. She had gotten away, and in her case it meant she had another chance to live due to the severity of the abuse that she endured. I was so happy to see that she had gotten her own apartment, and was back on her feet and there was such a sense of peace in her place that I wanted it, too. Tom was there with me and I believe that he knew that I had been awakened and that it was only a matter of time before I was going to leave him. He was right. I had made up my mind that very night when I saw my friend's happiness. I realized that I deserved to be happy, too.

When we returned home, I started packing, taking pictures off of the wall, and preparing myself to leave. I knew if I tried to kick him out, he would not go anywhere. He would always threaten to leave me, pack up his things and they would make it to the doorway, but he would never actually leave. This time, I did not want to give him the choice. I chose to leave. I continued to pack my things. My "Ah ha!" moment was here: the light bulb had come on and there was no putting it out!

I did not have any money to move, but I knew I had to do this; it had to be done now. So to get the money I needed, I refinanced the truck that Tom was driving (I bought it through my credit union). I was very direct with Tom: I told him I was going to refinance the truck so that I could get some money to move. He went along with it, not thinking I was serious, and even went with me to the finance company. He was there when I signed the contract to get the money. It took a day for me to pick up the check, so I guess Tom thought he had a little time to convince me to stay. He wasted no time to do so, and it went on for hours and hours. He became very agitated with me because I kept refusing to stay. In order for me to keep him calm, I pretended that I was going to stay.

The next morning, I went to work. I called the finance company and they told me that the check was ready for me to come pick up. I went on my lunch hour and picked up the check. When I got the check, I told the finance guy not to give out any information on the transaction. I went home after work and Tom was there. The first thing he told me was to call the finance company and tell them that I had changed my mind about the loan. I told I him that I would call them later, but he had got a business card the day before when he was with me. He called the manager of the company and told them that he was calling on behalf of me and that I had changed my mind about taking out the loan. They told him that I had already been down there and picked up the check. He became irate and screamed, "What!" He then threw the phone and started after me. I ran out the door and down the street. A Mexican family was outside sitting on their porch and their door was open, so I ran into their house. They did not speak English and I did not speak Spanish, but we communicated. They let me use their phone to call the police and hide in their house until the police came. While I was hiding in their house, I was looking out of the window and could see Tom riding down the street looking for me. He had a look on his face that I had never seen before and it scared me.

When the police came, I went back to the house. Tom was there and the police began their investigation. They put me in one room and him in another. Once we both told our sides, and I made it clear I wanted to leave, the police stayed so I could gather some of my things - mostly clothes. I left most of my personal things because I was focused on trying to get on with my life. The police made Tom move the truck so I could back my car out - he had blocked me in so I could not leave. So again, I was leaving all the things I worked hard for to preserve my safety.

Thankfully, a co-worker from the supermarket who knew my situation began to help me out. He told me that a man like Tom would not allow me to just up and leave him without a real fight. He allowed me to begin bringing small amounts of clothes and personal items over to his place and I stayed with him briefly as I searched for an apartment. Although this guy provided me with shelter when I needed it most, he was no saint. He was a hustler and a gambler, and he stole the money that I had set aside for my new apartment. He stole my saving bonds, he pawned my diamond ring, and he even took very precious family memorabilia, such as silver coins that I had been saving over the years that my dad had given me. Each time he did this, I had to go pay tons of fees to retrieve my jewelry from the pawn shop. He did this while I was at work so he could support his various habits. When I finally had saved up some money and an apartment I was looking at became available, I moved out into my own place again.

Months later, I reflected on my time with Tom and the things I had been through, and I became so upset about leaving my things with a man for the second time. I called my ex-partner Marcus and told him what happened with Tom. It had been over four years since I seen or talked to Marcus. I told him that I was going to get my gun and go back to the house where Tom was and I was going to get all of my things because I was not going to let another man take my things. Marcus could hear how upset I was and he told me not to worry about it, as he still had the furniture that I left with him five years ago and that I could come get it.

Marcus had put the furniture in storage. When I went to get it out, I found that a bill was due - he had not told me he was a month behind on his storage bill and was about to lose the contents. Nevertheless, I was glad to get the furniture back and counted my blessings. I had found an apartment and it was ready for me to move in with my reclaimed belongings. Thank God I had my beautiful furniture for my beautiful new apartment.

Shortly after I moved into my new apartment, my mom came to town. We went over to Tom's house, and my mom made him give me all of my things back, which I then put into storage. I was finally able to enjoy my freedom and my new apartment. And I had a blast!

The next relationship I found myself in was with Eric a few years later, after I moved back to Birmingham. I met Eric when I was traveling with a stage play. He was a set designer and also worked with the play. We became friends and went out together when we were touring different cities. We hung out when we were not working, as we had a lot in common. He never seemed to have any money so I would always pick up the tab. The first time he got paid, we went out to eat and he said "every man for himself." I should have left him alone then. I was picking up the tab the whole time we were hanging out, and he did not even offer to pay the tab when he got paid. When we were off the road and were not working, he would come to visit me in Birmingham and I would visit him in Atlanta. After many months of traveling back and forth from Birmingham to Atlanta, he asked me to move to Atlanta. I gave up my home in Birmingham and moved to Atlanta, and we found an apartment that we both liked.

Eric's sense for business was non-existent. One time, we went to Birmingham to build a set for a guy who was doing a stage play there. Eric's role was to build the sets and I was to do the makeup for the performers. Ultimately, Eric did not get paid for his work, but I did. I warned him not to put up the set before he got paid, but he did not listen to me and got screwed. He had brought a friend with us from Atlanta to help him build the set and because Eric did not get paid, I ended up having to use my money to pay his helper.

I worked with Eric in his shop, but that did not last long because of his questionable business practices. I got a job with Bronner Brothers and worked there a little over a year. I then opened my own Kiosk in Atlanta's West End Mall. About the same time, Eric fell ill after coming home from a set-building project in Alaska. He developed a blood clot in his leg and his health started to deteriorate. Before Eric's health began to fail, we were in the process of closing on a house. Eric was admitted to the hospital and learned that his leg would have to be amputated. He tried to keep this information from the people who were assisting with the house closing, but they ended up coming to the hospital so they could finish the paperwork to do the closing. Eric thought that he was going to get some money at the closing, but to his surprise they required more money from him to make the deal go through and I gave it to him.

It is funny: Eric was adamant that my name not be on the deed. I participated in the selection of the house and ultimate purchase, but Eric did not want me to have any ownership in it. I remember being so angry about it, but looking back, it was the best thing in the world that I was not on the deed to Eric's house because a year later I was able to buy my own.

Eric got out of the hospital after the amputation and needed almost around the clock assistance. The around the clock assistance was me. I helped him to get around, I changed his bandages, dumped his urine cups... everything. Thankfully, I had the help of one of his friends who came during the day while I was at work. Months went by and Eric got better, so much so that he felt up for a visit to his family in Florida. He did not take any of his urine cups with him. When Eric got back, I asked him how he managed without the urine cups. He told me that he went to the bathroom on his own. I said, "Well you gonna go to the bathroom on your own from now on, I won't be dumping another urine cup!" That conversation made me realize Eric could take care of himself, and freed me to move on with my life. I began preparing myself to move. I could not believe how selfish Eric was; I did so much for him and he appreciated it so little.

Eric was selfish, a taker not a giver, truly a mean person. He was a booster, a boaster and a procrastinator. He talked a big game about things he would do, but sat around and did very little if any of it. Although he had his own business - he was a set designer - and was extremely good at what he did, he was also slow, unorganized, and put things off until the last minute, which would then become a "rush-rush situation." But he had a purpose in my life. And although most of our connection was negative, I knew from past experience that there was something positive to learn and take away. The "good" that came from this bad situation was meeting Tyler Perry.

Eric was one of the first Black set designers in the 1990's in Atlanta. He designed and built sets for people who were in the entertainment business, including Tyler Perry. He is the reason that I met Tyler Perry back when Tyler was just getting started. Eric would build and store Tyler's play sets in his studio, The 11th Hour. Sometimes, Tyler would come there and rehearse for his plays, so I saw him going in and out all of the time. I was always working in the studio with Eric, painting and assisting him with the building of the sets. One day, while Tyler was there, I asked him if I could work with him doing make up for his plays. He said, "I don't have a budget for a makeup artist. If you come work with me, you'll have to do everything like unloading the trucks, helping with set up, working back stage with wardrobe or whatever else needs to be done." I said, "Okay," and left it at that.

I met up with Tyler Perry again years later, after he had made it big. I heard that he was doing a play at the Atlanta Civic Center and went backstage to meet him. I met him there since I already worked that venue. At first Tyler did not recognize me, but when I reminded him that we met previously at Eric's studio, he immediately remembered me. He said, "Oh, girl that's you? You clean up well. Every time I used to see you, you were covered in paint!"

I was so happy for Tyler. He had made it big! All of his hard work had paid off and I was seeing right in front of my face the fruits of his labor. He had gone from a jalopy to a Mercedes, and from selling his media products out the trunk of his car to having a packed house at the Civic Center to see his plays. This was amazing.

During our meeting, I patted his face (he had gained weight). I said to him, "You are looking good, you have gained weight." He said, "I'm eating now, when you knew me, I wasn't eating." I told him how great he looked and that "success agrees with you." He had on a cashmere jacket and I was just so proud that he had come such a long way from the last time that I had seen him as a struggling producer.

We laughed and talked and he then introduced me to one of his staff members, telling her that anytime that I wanted to come out to see a play to give me free tickets. I was a regular at his plays and met his mother once. At *"Woman Tho Art Loosed"*, a well known stage play, Tyler took me backstage and introduced me to the visionary and producer, Bishop TD Jakes and his wife Serita, Coretta Scott King (the wife of the famous Civil Rights Leader Dr. Martin Luther King Jr.), and their daughter Bernice King. During the introductions, I ran into my old friend Delilah Williams. I was so excited to see Delilah that I ran off to hug and talk to her. I had not seen her in years, since the times that we worked together on other stage plays. It amazes me how life comes full circle. At this time in our lives, we reunited backstage because I was with Tyler Perry who had become a household name and she was working with the world renowned Bishop TD Jakes on his project.

I would have loved to join Tyler as his makeup artist at that time, but I had just opened a new shop, renovated it, and had a five year lease obligation. However, after my lease ended, I turned my attention to getting back into the entertainment industry. I began to send out my resume to production companies. Patrice Coleman, the department head for Make Up at Tyler Perry Studios responded to my inquiry. She liked my work and came to my shop and looked at my portfolio. She then invited me to do make up for the set of *"I Can Do Bad All By Myself,"* *"Meet the Browns,"* and *"House Of Payne."* This is how I got started working with Tyler Perry. My first day on the set of *"I Can Do Bad All By Myself"*, I was working on Marvin Winans and Tyler happened to see me as he was directing the scene with Marvin and Gladys Knight. He came over and hugged me and said, "Long time," I responded, "It has been."

It was only later that I realized just what a divine connection had been made. I looked back through my contact cards and noticed an envelope with Patrice Coleman's name and address on it from when I was living in

Birmingham, long before I actually met her in person. Neither of us knew how her info came into my possession, but I know God's divine intervention when I see it. His direction, guidance, and favor make things happen that you can never do with your own knowledge or power. I give Him all the glory for the divine connections that He has made for me over the years, and He continues to order my steps to my place of destiny. I am very thankful for God's love towards me and His friendship along my journey. He is truly my best friend. He is more than a friend, He is my all and without Him I could not do anything. I am amazed at His thoughtfulness towards me to construct my life in such a way that I know without a doubt that He has been walking with me every step of the way. It warms my heart that I am in the center of His will and He continues to reward me with kindness, grace and supernatural blessings. God is an awesome God!

The early years...

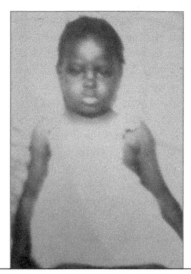

I was my dad's little "Peach Pie"!

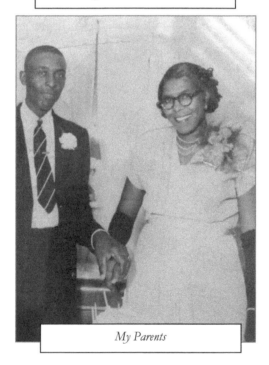

My Parents

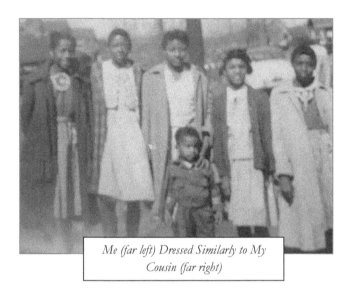

*Me (far left) Dressed Similarly to My
Cousin (far right)*

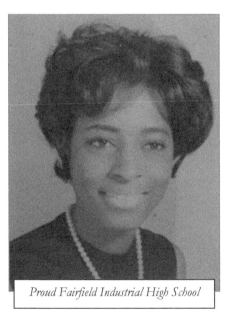

Proud Fairfield Industrial High School

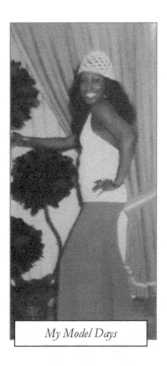

My Model Days

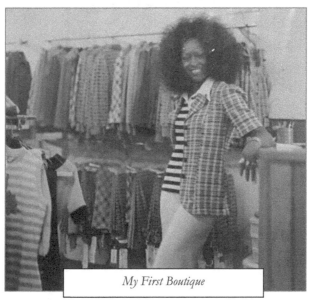

My First Boutique

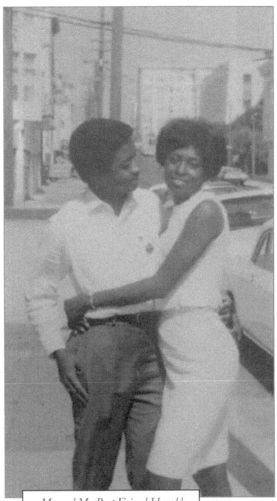

Me and My Best Friend Harold

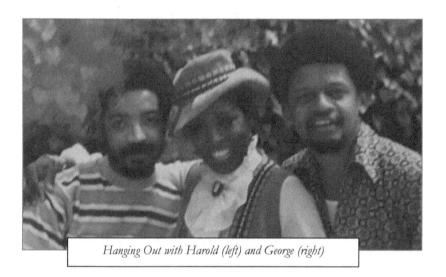

Hanging Out with Harold (left) and George (right)

A few pictures of my beautiful boutique.

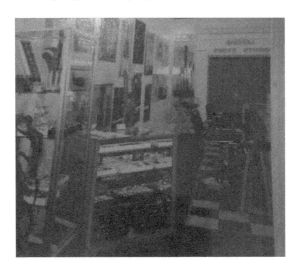

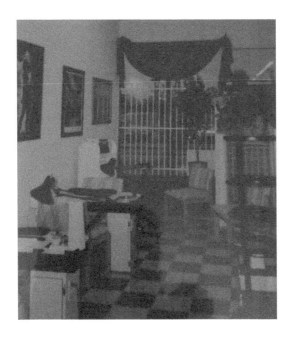

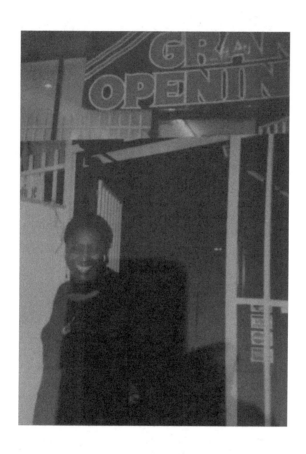

My time at the Masquers Club was amazing! The people I met, the things I learned, and the skills I acquired have blessed me in so many ways I cannot event count.

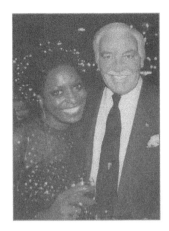 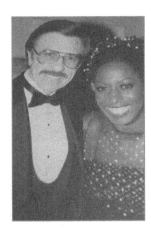

With Ceasar Romero (left) and Dan Rowan (right)

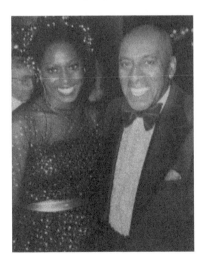

With Scatman Crothers

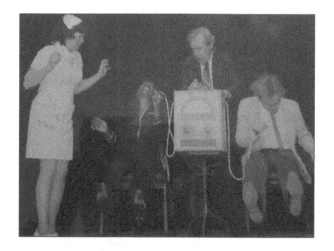

Having a great time during a comedy skit

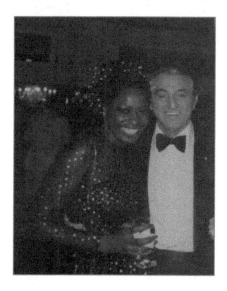

With Danny Thomas

Duke Ellington was so gracious. I keep this signed program as a momento of my wonderful time in Miami.

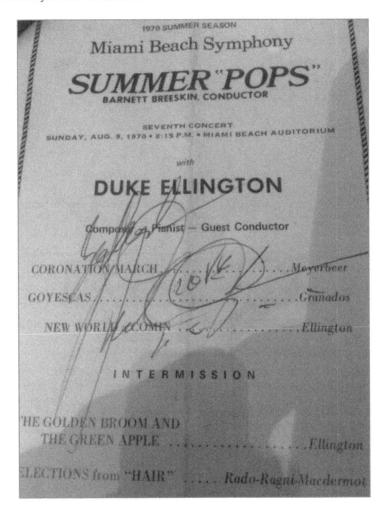

Sammy Davis, Jr., was a fantastic performer and gracious man.

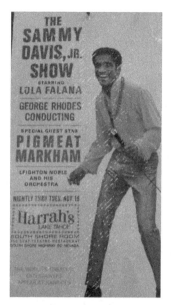

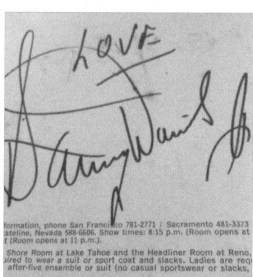

I really enjoyed sharing my Le Sure Dupre' makeup line with the world, and am preparing for the re-launch - stay tuned!

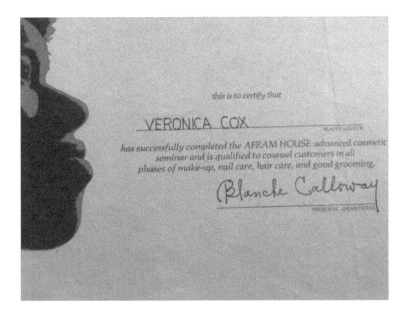

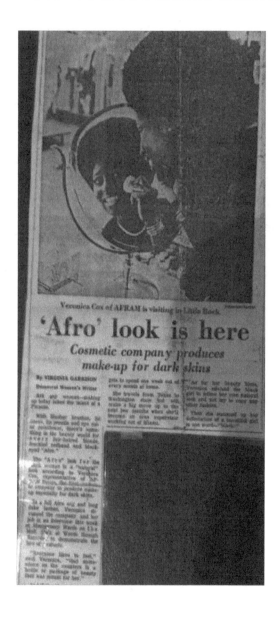

Veronica Cox of AFRAM is visiting in Little Rock.

'Afro' look is here
Cosmetic company produces make-up for dark skins

A Fort Worth STAR-TELEGRAM   Thursday Evening, May 27, 1976

Black Cosmetics

Bored, She Found a New, Fascinating Job

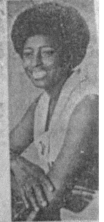

Veronica Lake Cox got bored with her job as a secretary for a San Francisco insurance company and started looking for something different.

She found it in the form of a new cosmetics firm, Afram House, which specializes in products made especially for the nation's 22 million black consumers.

That was a year ago, and the longest time she has stayed "put" in any one state in that time is the week she is spending in Dallas, and the week in Fort Worth. She will be at the Montgomery Ward store at Riverside and Berry streets for the rest of this week. Sharon Martin, another representative of Afram, is at the Seventh Street Montgomery Wards.

* * *

VERONICA explained that Afram, Inc., is headed by Miss Blanche Calloway, sister of Cab Calloway and a former actress herself. Blanche Calloway found that makeup artists in the theater never were able to properly make up her dark skin.

She began to work with a chemist to manufacture the right cosmetics for dark skin, and the result is the Afram line. Miss Calloway believes that cosmetics are a part of equal rights. "Today, there is no limit for a woman of color. She is competing for jobs that

cosmetics firm, Veronica Cox makes up white women as well as black women. "In some cities, almost all your customers are white," she said.

The black cosmetics differ in consistency and in color. Eyeshadows, for instance, are generally lighter and heavier than those designed for white complexions. False eyelashes in the line are curlier, because a black woman's eyelashes naturally are curlier than those of white women.

Pink or red lipsticks are "too bright for black skin." Miss Cox recommends the frosted whites for young women, and the very dark, almost black, lipsticks for older women.

* * *

LIKE MISS Calloway, Miss Cox has a theatrical background. She went to Los Angeles from her native Birmingham to attend theatrical school, decided she couldn't live in Los Angeles, and left after six months to make her home in San Francisco.

Later on, she found that the producer of the movie "Kiss and Kill" had been hunting her in Los Angeles to offer her a role in the movie. She felt she had missed a great opportunity—until she saw the movie.

Recently an assignment took Veronica Cox close

—Star-Telegram Photo
VERONICA COX

65

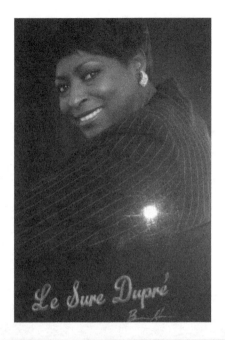

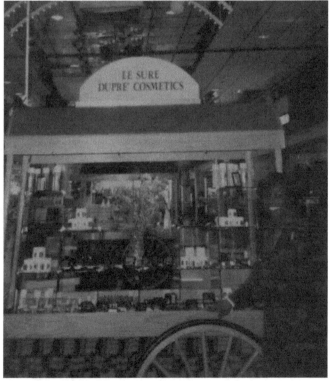

My time in Brazil with Harold and his friends was unbelievable! The dinner parties, outings, and fantastic people I encountered were incredible!

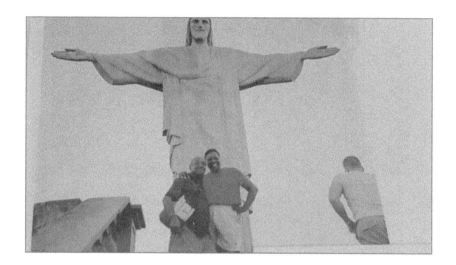

I am so blessed! I have worked with and met some talented and committed people!

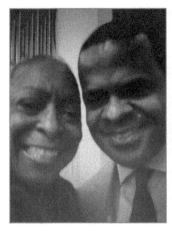 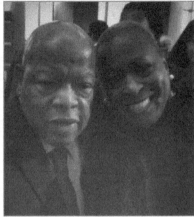

With Atlanta Mayor Kasim Reed (left) and Civil Rights icon US Congressman John Lewis (right)

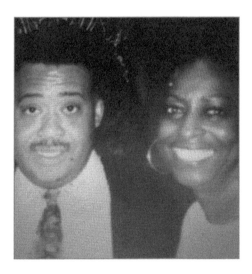

With Rev. Al Sharpton

My time during the Civil Rights Movement was a mixture of pride, pain, hope, fear, and love. I was humbled and overwhelmed when I was recognized for my leadership by various organizations as a "Foot Soldier for Freedom".

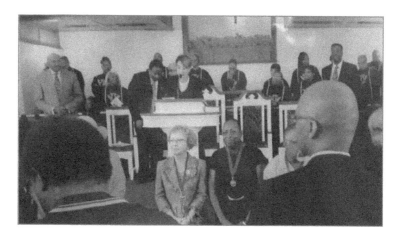

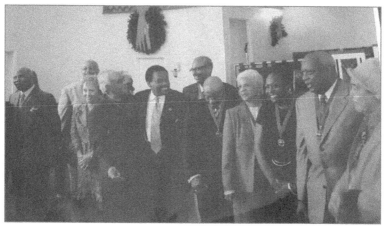

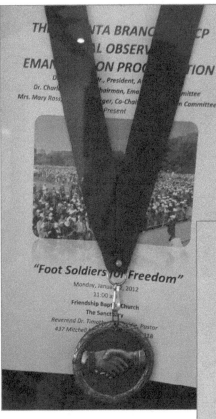

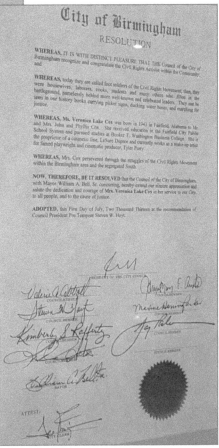

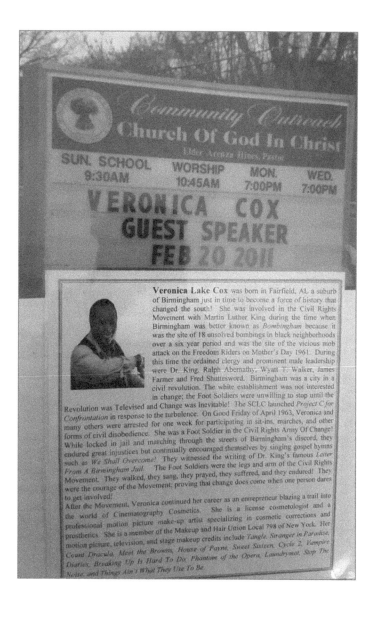

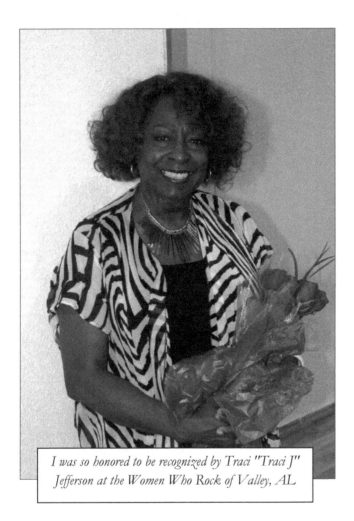

I was so honored to be recognized by Traci "Traci J" Jefferson at the Women Who Rock of Valley, AL

My God children are my heart, truly the apples of my eye.

I still cannot believe my sweet Angel Alison is gone, but I know she rests with the Lord now.

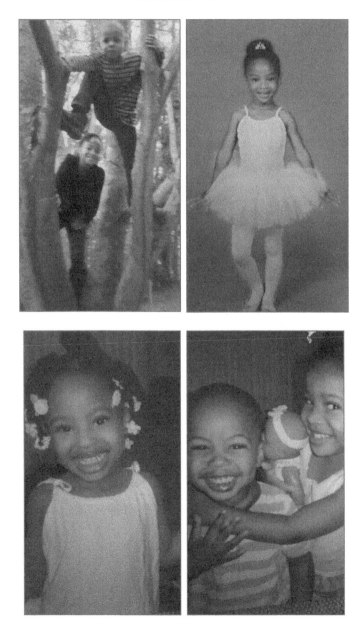

CHAPTER 9

MY BEST FRIEND

Harold was my best friend. Even when I was very young, I knew that he was special and would be a special part of my life.

Harold grew up two doors down from me, and his mother had all the boys and my mother had all the girls: every time my mother had a girl, his mother had a boy. Every time us kids got together and played "house," Harold and I were always husband and wife.

I really did not like food, but my mom made it a requirement that I eat before I could go outside and play. Harold knowing this would help me out by making my dinner "disappear." He would then call my mom and let her know that I had eaten all of my food so we could play together. How I loved my friend. When I think about him, all I have are happy thoughts, good thoughts. He was an escape from the hell that I experienced at home. I always looked forward to seeing him come up to the house so that we could play together. If he was not visiting my house, I was visiting his. We loved playing together. We had so much fun. I actually used to get a bit upset when he would have to leave and go visit his grandparents for weeks at a time during the summer. I used to wonder why his other siblings did not spend as much time visiting their grandparents... I would miss Harold so much while he was gone and I felt abandoned while he was away. He always lifted me up and he told me that I could do anything. He showed me a different way of living, a better side of life, and excitement. He often told me how valuable I was and how I needed to recognize my own self worth. Next to my dad, he was the most significant male in my life. This nurturing connection with Harold helped me to believe in myself more, and not to accept the negative things that others would say about me. He was always boosting me up and giving me hope.

Harold was everything a good friend should be. He taught me a lot. He taught me about proper etiquette, even the proper way to eat. I could talk to him about anything, even the things that I could not talk to my sisters or other family members about, I could always share with Harold.

There was an old man in our neighborhood who used to call Harold my husband because we were together so much. It seems that I have always known him as far back as I can remember. He has always been there. He was like a family member, closer than a brother, closer than my own siblings.

Coming up together during our high school years, Harold sometimes helped me with my homework. In eighth or ninth grade, he had a crush on one of my friends, Gloria. She was beautiful and a very sweet girl. He had me going back and forth playing matchmaker between them. It was so sweet. He was crazy about her! Harold and Gloria dated throughout high school. Shortly after we graduated,

Harold tried to plan a birthday gift for her (her birthday was coming up in September). I called her to try to get some information about what she might like for her birthday, only to find that Gloria had moved to LA. She had not told anyone that she was moving, not even Harold. When Harold got the news, he ran down to her house looking for her, but she was long gone. This hurt him to his heart. He later dated another girl while in college, but it did not compare to the love that he had for Gloria. She left a hole in his heart that was never filled.

After college, Harold reconnected with Gloria. She had two children and was married to an abusive husband. I talked to Gloria, and she told me, and later Harold, that her mother made her go to California and told her not to tell Harold because if he wanted her bad enough he would come after her.

Harold graduated from high school, then went to Wilberforce University in Ohio. He could not stay there because his folks could not afford to keep him there. As a result, he came back home to Birmingham and continued his education at Miles College in Fairfield, suburbs of Birmingham. While at Miles, he pledged Omega Psi Phi Fraternity, Inc., was president of the Junior Class and President of the Student Body his senior year. He travelled all over Birmingham and parts of Alabama representing Miles College with other college officials. I was able to go with him sometimes. I went with them so much on their college tours that I felt that I also was a Miles College representative.

At this time, I was a student at Booker T. Washington Business College and got involved in the Civil Rights Movement during the years of 1963 and 1964. After the movement, I dropped out of school and moved to New York. This was about the same time Harold returned home from Wilberforce.

I came back home around 1965. In 1966, Harold graduated from Miles College and moved to San Francisco because of a new job opportunity at San Francisco State University. When he told me about it, I was so excited for him, but at the same time I was not happy that he was leaving me. He quickly reminded me that I had left him when I moved to New York.

When Harold had been in San Francisco about a year, I called to tell him that I needed to get away from Birmingham immediately due to the problems that I was having at home with my mom. He told me to come to San Francisco. I was relieved, as we had never been away from each other for such long periods of time. My mom did not want me to go, but I went anyway of course. I had to find out what life was like away from home. I had to take a chance and pursue my dreams. And Harold was right there with me!

When I moved to San Francisco, Harold had all kinds of things for us to do, and everybody loved him. Harold was very intelligent and always organized. He was just a beautiful person. You could not meet a better, more honest person than Harold. He would tell you what he felt, good or bad. I remember when I got my first job in

San Francisco. I was all nervous and scared, and he said, "You gotta get out here. You can't be up in here like this. You gotta get out there and find out what bus is running and what time it comes and goes. You gotta call these places and find out how to get to them." I remember wanting to literally regurgitate hearing all the things I had to do, but he just kept on saying, "You're a grown woman now; you gotta come on with it." So I learned from him and I wound up preaching the same message to family members who came to stay with me as they ventured away from home to get a new start. I would tell them that they had to "get up and get at it" and take the bull by the horns and be proactive about making progress in their lives.

With my first paycheck, I secured my very first apartment. Harold was a bit upset with me because he was not present when I got the apartment. He wanted to make sure that it was a safe place and that everything was good for me. Thankfully it was and Harold was pleased with my new place.

Harold introduced me to so many people, especially his fraternity brothers. The house was always full of the brothers of Omega Psi Phi. They had an Omega House in San Jose, and we spent a lot of time there. The girlfriends of the Omegas were called the QTs; because I would hang out partying with the Omegas and their girlfriends, I was also considered a QT. Harold's roommate, Carl, was the Basileus (or president) of the Fraternity, so they hosted all kinds of outings, and it was never a dull moment with them.

Harold moved to Redwood City to be closer to his new job at Stanford University. I moved down in the peninsula with him, but got my own place shortly after. Not too long after moving to Redwood City, Harold met a new friend named George. Harold took me over to George's house to introduce me to his new friend. At that time I did not know what was going on between the two of them. Looking back, I remember it being funny that George had more décor items than I had. His kitchen was laid out with all kinds of gadgets, he had sets of everything, and his taste was impeccable. I was impressed with all of George's gourmet displays and made a joke that his kitchen looked better than mine - or any other woman that I knew for that matter. We all laughed and went on to enjoy a beautiful evening.

Weeks later, Harold called me and told me he wanted to come over to talk with me. He said he *really* had something to tell me. He came over and we went walking through the streets of San Francisco. Harold shared that he in fact was gay and that George was his love interest. I replied to him, "AND?" I was a bit upset because he had me all anxious that he was going to tell me something drastic. I was relieved that it was not something more serious and he was relieved that I still loved and accepted him just as he was. He was now openly comfortable with his homosexuality. I could never see him any differently because he was like my right arm. I was just happy that he had come into his own and was happy being who he was. A few months later, Harold moved from Redwood City back to San Francisco to be with George.

Harold and George exposed me to so many other cultures and international customs. They would have these full day parties where many of their friends were invited to take part in cooking and creating art pieces. George never bought bread; he baked it fresh. Some of his friends from Berkley, and other prestigious schools, who loved to experiment with recipes would come over and make the best gourmet dishes. Others who were more interested in arts and crafts would gather outside on the patio or in other parts of the house while the chefs were preparing our dishes for the grand feast to come. We all would have our butter ready to taste-test the breads as they were prepared; you could smell the aroma all over the house. I joined the arts and crafts folks, and we made candles, home decorations and reinvented cultural artifacts. When the food was ready, Harold and the other chefs would call us all in to eat... it was like a great feast! Then we would party all night and enjoy each other's company. I was truly blessed to have met Harold's friends - they became my friends and my new family. I can honestly say that those were *the best* years of my life! I have not felt that blessed since then. Being surrounded by such love was pure bliss.

When I say that I was able to experience pure bliss and was surrounded by love, literally I was. In addition to having the love of my best friend, his friends that became my friends, better yet family, I also was in San Francisco during the Hippie Movement. This movement was started by rich young white kids who were basically rebelling against their parents who they considered The Establishment. They joined together to make several statements to the world: we have our own thoughts, we do not have to accept the racist beliefs and behaviors of our families and forefathers; we are one, a colorless generation; we love everyone and are not afraid to show it; and we will show love to the world and make a difference for good. That is why they were called the Flower Children: they wanted to show the world that all people are beautiful no matter their color.

The Hippie's beliefs were exemplified by the clothes they wore: although these kids were often very privileged and had access to money, their clothes were usually an expression of the opposite. They would put on whatever felt comfortable. I laugh now because thinking back, lots of their outfits looked like rags of many colors that were thrown together haphazardly; but they were happy and not caught up in the materialistic things of the world. This was another statement that the Hippie Generation made.

I remember when I first got to San Francisco and was introduced to this movement. I had just come from a small town in the South where everyone in my community looked the same, just like me. We felt the oppression of Jim Crow laws and were extremely segregated from the whites. So when I got to San Francisco and saw the streets full of all of these white kids, mixed with blacks kids, and Latinos, and Asians hanging out together, hugging each other, even working and living together, I was absolutely in awe. It was such a beautiful site and so different from everything that I had known growing up back in Alabama.

The Golden Gate Park area was a famous gathering place for the Hippies. There was always music playing and concerts in the park. People would sit around with all kinds of instruments making their own music. They had flutes, guitars, drums and they all just played away. No matter what time it was, day or night, there were traffic jams of sight seers driving by, just to catch a glimpse of these young kids who were expressing their true freedom. Literally, it was normal to see people naked, sunbathing, making love under their blankets or in the bushes in the park. They were enjoying life on their own terms, spreading joy and happiness. They also enjoyed nature's gift of marijuana. There was so much "Mary Jane" being smoked in that area that you would get an immediate contact high from just being there.

I do not recall seeing any police in the area during the Hippie Movement. I guess there was no cause for their presence as everyone was at peace. There was no fighting, arguing or anything of the sort. It was such a peaceful atmosphere; there was no fear of anyone stealing from you, hurting you, or being violent at all. There was just peace and love in the air… and marijuana of course!

It was so funny to me- it seemed like every Hippie had two things: a flower somewhere on their person and a dog. Even when they used public transportation, their dogs would ride the bus with them. The strange part to me was that the dogs had to pay a full fare to ride the bus! So, their owners paid their full fare, the dogs sat down in their seats and rode the bus like people. If you were to get on a bus and a dog had taken the last seat, you would just have to stand up as the dog paid for his right to sit and travel.

I was a part of this movement. I went to work during the day, got off, changed into my Hippie gear and hung out in the park with everyone else. I walked the streets and browsed the shops along Haight and Ashbury. This area, "The Haight Ashbury" area, was known to be a Hippie community. Thinking back, I felt so happy to have been a part of this era. It was truly a highlight of my life; the San Francisco Hippie era. I have not experienced such peace, happiness and joy at that level since. The mindsets of the people during this time completely changed my perspective about life. It made me more aware of the blessings of being alive and having what some would call, "the small things" in life (that are not so small), like friends and love. They really demonstrated the importance of fully embracing who you are and being that person in spite of what others may think. Hippies embodied the now well known statement, "Do You," meaning be your own person, do what comes natural to you, and live without limitations. I loved that no one judged during this time. No one was concerned about materialism and there was no competition with others. That was so refreshing.

God had again put me in the right place at the right time. This seemed to be a pattern for me as God positioned me to be a part of real-life American History. The first time was when I was part of the Civil Rights Movement in Birmingham and the second was being part of the Hippie Movement. The third was when I lived in Los Angeles and Atlanta during the Olympics (1984 and 1996, respectively). How many people can say that they lived in all of these places and literally were a part of all of these historic moments and movements in our country? Not many I am sure, but I was and I am truly blessed.

Two years after my glorious Hippie experience, I moved to LA, but of course I visited San Francisco - and Harold - often. When I visited Harold, he and his friends took great care of me. They were beautiful people who looked out for me as if I was their little sister. When Harold was at work or not able to be with me due to his schedule, I was always entertained: I had a lunch date every day with one of Harold's friends. And every night, we had amazing dinner parties, alternating houses between Harold and his friends. We had the time of our lives. Classy, elegant, fabulous, and extraordinary examples of people with genuine hearts, our friends knew how to treat people. They were kind, honest, caring, loving and pure. They always had formal dinners with wine and candlelight. Everything they did, they did with class. They would dress in furs and take limousines to theaters. They took me in as their own and went out of their way to show me the life of the rich and famous: good food, good wine and other delicacies. Harold's friends enjoyed the finer things in life and I got used to enjoying that lifestyle because of them. I so enjoyed going to the operas, theaters, plays and Broadway musicals. I remember George having to translate the musicals that were in Latin so that I would understand what was going on.

At one point, Harold and George decided they wanted to travel the world. They sold everything they had and toured the world for three years. They bought a brand new Volkswagen van and picked it up in Germany. They drove all over Europe and, if they couldn't drive, they would ship the van to the next country they were destined to visit. They did this until the money ran out.

At the end of their journey, Harold and George went to New Orleans where George's family lived to make some decisions about their life, where they would go from there. George wanted to begin to cater, using his cooking skills, and live his dreams in San Francisco. However, Harold did not want to return to the lab at Stanford, so he began searching the newspaper for other opportunities that would allow him to continue traveling the world.

Harold found an opening with Trans World Airlines (TWA). He was hired immediately and sent to New York to begin this new job. Harold spent over 30 years with TWA. He started at the entry level and became the company's top flight attendant. Harold spoke four languages: French, Spanish, English and Portuguese. He was the guy who made the announcements during international flights. TWA created a specialized plaque in Harold's honor "Top International Flight Attendant" that was displayed on an airplane that flew everywhere... and it had his name on it!

I cannot say enough how smart Harold was. He was absolutely brilliant. While working at the airline, he was chosen to take care of the Pope when he travelled to the US from The Vatican. Harold was the only one chosen to be the Pope's Personal Assistant when the airline flew him back to The Vatican.

After Harold had been working with the airline for about fifteen years, George met someone else - Timmy. Harold was generally always away in flight, so he and George became roommates while Timmy and George became an item. Harold started dating other people, too, and he and George remained friends as well as roommates.

Although Harold met other great guys, their relationships just never compared to his relationship with George. Sadly, Timmy contracted AIDS and passed away, and about a year or two later, George also became very sick with the virus. Harold cared for him until he passed away.

Things were going well with Harold, but then he contracted Hepatitis. He almost died but for a friend of his who worked for Jet Blue. He called Harold one day and noticed Harold was irrational; he was talking "out of his head," so he went to check on him. When he arrived, he saw Harold was really sick and in bad condition. He grabbed Harold and carried him to the hospital. Harold was definitely at the point of death and God sent an angel, his friend, by his house to save him. A few years after Harold's recovery, this same friend who saved his life ended up losing his in an airplane that went down in the Florida Everglades. As far as I know, the plane got buried in the swamp and they were never able to get it out. This was quite disturbing to Harold, not only that the friend that saved his life died, but the way he died was tragic. Harold was never able to get closure as there was no body, no final goodbye. Harold continued as a flight attendant. I am sure the thoughts of his friend's tragic death by plane crash shook him often, but he held up well through the ordeal and still remained a source of strength for others in the years to come.

A mutual friend of ours who we had known for many years during our time living in San Francisco. This friend later moved to Brazil, and Harold spent a significant amount of time there. My first visit to Brazil, our friend arranged a dinner party for me on my first night and it was beautiful. I did not know it at the time, but Harold planned my entire trip - everything - out to the last detail. He even subleased an apartment while I was there.

Harold was well cultured and well traveled. Every night we went to a different restaurant. The food was excellent and Harold told me he was saving the best restaurant for last, but I could not imagine food being better than what I already had.

We went to the Christ and to Sugarloaf and several other places. Harold had museum and theater tickets ready for me. He rented a car and a driver, and took me to all of the historical places in Rio.

The mornings were something to remember with Harold in Brazil. In Brazil, they grind fresh coffee beans every day, so Harold got fresh coffee for us every morning along with fresh bread. He even warmed the milk for our coffee and he always had cloth napkins. (You would never catch him with a paper napkin.)

One of the most beautiful memories that I have about Brazil with my friend is after breakfast time, we would stroll and enjoy the tropical scenery. There were these coconut stands where the natives would chop off the top of the coconut for us, place a straw in them and we enjoyed fresh coconut milk while sitting on the beach watching the ocean. What a magnificent sight.

Harold was always back and forth to Brazil. It was like a second home for him. He said once that he did not have to travel to any other countries because he had basically seen the entire world and had found his heaven on earth in Brazil.

While on a visit, Harold met a special guy and they later became an item. He seemed to be excited about this new love relationship. I honestly feel that Harold was possibly more into him than he was into Harold, as later Harold found out that his guy was not faithful to him. Harold set his friend up in an apartment and would visit on occasion. On a surprise visit he got surprised himself as he found another man there and it looked as if they were in a relationship. It crushed him. I believed that this was one of the triggers to his battle with depression. Unfortunately, he was never able to bounce back from this episode. So many things had begun to pile upon him and the weight was unbearable. It seemed like a downward spiraling of tragic life events that caused Harold to sink deeper and deeper into a depression that he just could not shake.

Around the same time that Harold was betrayed by his lover in Brazil, his house in New York caught on fire and he did not have any insurance. Thankfully, his friends threw him a party at a club to help raise money to take care of his immediate needs. That was also around the time when he was feeling low from being disrespected at his job, losing his seniority, and being bossed around by new young people who had little to no experience with the new airline that he was working with. They were a local airline and he was used to flying internationally. With this local airline, they gave him a hard time on a daily basis and the job that he used to love had become a major source of frustration for him. Harold felt like he had accomplished so much as a 30 year veteran in the industry with tons of experience and professional accolades. He spoke several languages and had spent so much of his life in the industry as a top seasoned international flight attendant. Now, he had been transitioned to a local airline and was being tossed aside, bossed around, and mistreated by people who could not come anywhere near his professional resume. This was an insult to his manhood, being constantly devalued at the workplace.

I saw Harold go through some hard times in his life: major relationship failures, career challenges, and financial problems; but I never knew the extent of the hurt and pain that he was suffering. Harold always tried to hide his true emotions by

81

keeping a "happy face" on for the public, wanting everyone to believe everything was okay in his life. His suicide came as a shock to me, but I had started feeling something different about him a month or so before he died. Really, before that because he was working for TWA for about 30 years when the airline merged. Instead of him retiring like most of his coworkers, he went on with the new company. They used him for two years, kicked him to the curb, and Harold had to start all over again.

At one point, I remember Harold was so depressed that he took off from his job, stating that he was sick. He took a company flight to stay with his brother while in DC. When the airline found out that had taken a flight during the time that he was ill, he was scolded. They said that if he was sick that he should not be flying, he should be at home recovering. Harold was furious and that was it for him. He ranted to me and his brother that those folks could take their "Mickey Mouse job" and shove it.

Harold continued to stay with his brother for a while, and he noticed Harold was just not himself. He would stay in bed all day, often curled up in the fetal position. This went on for a while, then Harold left and went back home to New York to stay with a long time friend. She opened her house to him when his home burned down. She was not only a close friend and confidant, she was Harold's wife.

Harold trusted me a lot; so much so that he hassled me for years to marry him so I could take advantage of his benefits, such as health insurance and the privileges of flying together as a married couple. He wanted to protect me and also did not want those benefits to go to waste. I declined, as I wanted to leave myself open for marriage. His mother had passed away and less than two years later, his dad died. They used to fly with him and made use of those benefits, too. Harold approached me again about marriage, as he wanted me to get the benefits since both of his parents were gone. He begged me for years and I just would not do it. His (then-future) wife, who was friend to us both, accepted the proposal and it worked out for the both of them.

Weeks after Harold got back to New York he attempted suicide by drinking antifreeze and passed out in Central Park. Someone found him and got him to the hospital in time to save his life. However, he was in a comma for a while, then released to the psychiatric ward for two weeks. This was his first known suicide attempt.

I was living in Atlanta and running my business, so I could not go see Harold, but I called him after he came home from the hospital and told him how disappointed everyone would have been if he had been successful. He responded by saying that he had not thought about that. When Harold got out of the hospital, I was so very happy that he was still alive, and had high hopes that things would get better. I was glad I had not lost my dear friend.

Each year, we called each other on our birthdays without fail. That particular year, he had just been released from the psychiatric ward from his suicide attempt and called me to let me know that he had not forgotten about my birthday. He said that he just wanted me to know that he was still thinking about me. I called him on his birthday, which was two weeks later. He told me that he was still feeling anxious. I did not know what he meant by that. He had come into the house and answered the phone right when the machine was picking it up. He told me that we needed to get off the phone because he thought the machine was recording us. I thought that he was going to call me back, but he did not.

Less than 24 hours later, my friend stood in front of a New York subway train and killed himself. His wife was at work and no one was around. He did not leave any good-bye letters or anything; he just left us just like that.

After Harold's death, his wife told me that she sometimes found him in his room sitting in the dark and in total silence for days, and he would not come out. The illness had taken over and he could not come back from it.

Harold's death really hurt me. I was absolutely devastated when I heard the news. When my dad was killed, I was hurt of course, but his death was not at his own hands. This hurt was different, it was worse. I still get angry every time I think about it. I felt anger, disappointment, and hurt. You put this person on a pedestal all of your life and this is what they do to you? It was like someone took a knife and stuck it in my heart and just twisted and twisted it. I wish I could have done more. If there was anything that I could have done to prevent Harold's suicide, God knows that I would have. I really wish that I had understood what he meant when he told me that he felt anxious during our last conversation. A part of me died when Harold did. I had just talked to him and tried to encourage him, then the next day he killed himself. I was angry, confused, and lost because he was the major source of joy in my life.

Harold "came out of the closet" to me in our adulthood, but I was not surprised when he told me he was gay. I knew it all the time, and so did my family. He did not know it, but people in my family called him "Miss Harold" when he was not around. I am not sure how he did not know that we all knew that he was gay. When we played house as kids, we would argue over what the dolls would wear, who would dress them and style their hair. As a child, I never thought about society's gender roles or the fact that others perceived Harold as having feminine ways. I just enjoyed my friend's company and loved him for who he was. Obviously, Harold tried to fight against his natural feelings and played the straight role for many years before finally coming into his own, accepting who he was and living his life without restraints.

It is really eerie that one of Harold's college roommates, Walter, also committed suicide just a few years before Harold. They went to the same high school, graduated at the top of their classes with honors, and they were the top performers in their professions. They lived in the same community and had achieved most of their professional goals. They were both brilliant men who contributed so much to the world, but they both took their own lives. This goes to show you that no matter what you have going for yourself, be it riches, fame, a great education, or success; it does not bring you happiness. Regardless of your material wealth, fame, fortune, and even all of the worldly successes, those things cannot fulfill you. There is a fulfillment in life that only comes from being connected to God and being filled with His Spirit, joy and love. There is a supernatural peace that comes from having a strong faith in God, who is more powerful than you alone. If you do not have this deep rooting in God, it is very easy to be blown away by the trials and storms of life because you are not anchored properly in your Spiritual life. You must know without a shadow of a doubt that when your strength has ended, and you feel that you cannot go on, God will carry you through everything. A beautiful promise in God's Word says, "In your weakness, God's strength is made perfect." In other words, when you are the weakest, that is when God can be strong for you. But you must let go, and let God. In order to do that, you must have faith that God will be there for you. If you lose your faith, you lose everything. Never lose your faith in God's ability to get you through your storms and bring you out stronger by His power.

When my dearest friend Harold took his own life, it was almost too much for me to bear. I knew however, that through the grief and pain of losing him, I must move on with my life. I had to push past the pain and live my life. That is what Harold would have wanted me to do.

CHAPTER 10

HOMELESS BUT NOT HOPELESS

Ben was a casual friend who would come around from time to time, and we would go out occasionally. My mechanic introduced us. I was not expecting anything great to come from him, I just enjoyed his company. He ended up being a slick hustler just like the others. He stayed around long enough to hear about what I had and figured out how he could get his hands on it. I came into some money from a settlement and he was giving me advice on how to invest it and get greater returns. I did not get all the details on the investment deal, but I gave him $15,000 to invest. About the same time, I was planning to move from my apartment. I sued my landlord because he had not painted my place in the eight years I lived there. The judge told me I had a great case, but because I had not put the money in a special account for rent until the legal case was over, I lost. As a result, I had to move out of my apartment immediately. I was not worried because I knew that Ben was working on getting the returns from the investment. I was looking to buy a condo, and Ben convinced me that he could get a good return on my investment that I could use to put down on my purchase, thereby lowering my mortgage payments.

About the same time, I met a Jewish guy by the name of Joseph Rothstein on a beach at a bar restaurant. He was an older gentleman. We became friends and talked all the time over the phone and occasionally he took me out. I told him about losing the case in court and being evicted, and he offered his home to me so I could stay for a while. I placed all of my stuff in storage and continued to call Ben to check on the returns of the investment. Each time I called, he gave me one excuse after another. Finally, he told me that the money was gone. No other explanation. I asked him to meet me to explain, he agreed, but later changed his mind because he said that he knew that I carried a gun. He then threatened me saying that if we met and he saw me go into my purse (for the gun) that he would shoot me first. That was the last time that I heard from him. He changed his number and was nowhere to be found. It was like he fell off the face of the earth, and I did not know how to find him. Unfortunately, I did not know very much about Ben. I did not know where he lived and I did not get his license plate number when he would come visit. I had nothing to use to find him. I later found out that he had given me a false name, so he was not even who he said he was. I trusted him so much because he told me he was a police officer, but I actually never saw his badge. He told me that he did not show his badge often because people would call in and make false charges against him so I just took him at his word. When I reported that he had run off with my money to the police, I found out that he was not a police officer at all. The police told me that by law a police officer is supposed to show their badge. He had lied to me the whole time. Again, I had been taken advantage of by another man who proclaimed to care about me.

I called one of my brothers for help; he was a booster and boaster. He was the first Black police officer in Fairfield, Alabama. My mom spoiled him to no end. He was my mom's baby. According to my dad, his name was "sorry." My brother had his own barbeque business. Although his wife, two daughters, and other family members helped him make it work, he spent a lot of his money gambling. When he was not losing money at the track, the employees were stealing it from the cash register.

My brother boasted so much about his money. He bragged about being able to pay cash for his nice cars, keeping thousands of dollars in paper bags in his home, and being able to blow cash. It was really strange that my brother, who constantly bragged about his riches, could not or would not help me out of a tough situation that ultimately led me to be homeless. I called on my brother when I was going through a very tough time in LA. I needed money to pay my storage bill, get a place, and pay my last car note. He ended up calling all of my family members to collect money for me while telling everyone my business in the process. Instead of wiring me the money that I needed, he used some of the monies that he had collected on a plane ticket and flew out to LA where I was. He paid the storage bill and my car note, then gave me $100 and told me to spend it wisely. Then he flew his behind back to Alabama boasting to everyone back home about how he had helped me and taken care of business, when he actually left me, his sister, in LA basically homeless to fend for myself.

My Jewish friend Joe, who I had been living with for months, was now in the process of moving out of his apartment due to his emphysema (he needed a different climate to get better). I did not know what I was going to do. I had no clue where I was going to go after Joe moved. Joe was shocked and disappointed in the condition that my brother had left me, and in total disbelief my brother had done that. He had been waiting on my brother to get there because he was moving out the next day. When my brother left, I was crying because I did not know what I was going to do or where I was going. At that very moment the phone rang. It was my cousin's wife, who lived in West Covina, CA. She called at the exact time that I was asking God for help. I did not have a job or money, and my cousin and his wife took me in. They extended their home to me during my time of need and I was so grateful.

After staying in their home for a short period of time, I came to find out that she had real issues. I would awake early to go out looking for work or go on interviews and would get home pretty late some nights. At first, she would cook meals for the entire family and when I would return home from job hunting, I would go in the fridge and eat the leftovers. At some point, things changed and there were not any leftovers saved for me to eat. I took the hint and left my cousin's house and moved in with Greg, a person I met from church. He ended up kicking me out because I would not sleep with him. Imagine that. I was in a desperate situation, and was forced to call on an ex-boyfriend, Tom, for help. This ex had lots of anger issues and when we were together, had forced me to call the police on him while trying to get away from him. This was the guy who locked my things up and would not allow me access to my property after I left the relationship.

When I called to ask if I could stay with him for a few weeks, Tom was more than happy to oblige. I stayed with him for a very short while, maybe less than a month. He wanted us to get back together, but I told him that was not what I wanted. To top it off, he told me he had a girlfriend! She would come over from time to time during the week and on weekends. Sometimes when she came over during the week, I had to sleep in my car or if it was a weekend, in various places. Unfortunately, I got into a car accident and totaled my car, leaving me with no place to sleep but Tom's van. To sleep in Tom's van, I had to go outside and hide behind the bushes until the coast was clear for me to get into the van so people in the community would not see me. I would sleep in there until it was time for Tom to go to work, then I would go in the house after he and his girlfriend left. That got old very quickly, and a few weeks later, I got a rental car.

As soon as I could manage it, I moved from Tom's house to a condo where I rented a room from a young lady. I lived there a few months until I got a lump sum settlement. The accident that I had a few months earlier turned out to be a blessing in disguise, because I was rewarded enough money to get my own place. After I got my place, I went to get my furniture out of storage. Things seemed to be getting better... but when I got to the storage unit, my keys did not fit the lock. I had two units together and neither key worked, so I went to the office for them to come open the unit. I could not understand why my keys were not working. Although it had been over two months since I had checked on the unit, the last time I checked my keys worked. When the people from the office came out to help me, they cut the locks and walked away. They did not even take the locks off or open the doors to the units. They just walked away.

When the people from the moving company that I hired opened the doors to the units, and I saw that all of my things had been taken, I could not believe it; I thought I was having a bad dream. Everything had been stolen. I had been paying storage fees for several months, only to lose all my exquisite household furniture. It seemed like I could not win for losing! I took off running towards a busy street. I did not know what I was doing. I had lost my mind. The movers ran after me and caught me before I got into the street. It took me a while to pull myself together. But by the grace of God, I did pull myself together, took the few items that were left in my storage unit, and brought them to my new place. I decided to make do with what I had and become content with my situation. I made a plan to focus on the future, and started cosmetology school which helped me to keep my mind off the negatives and focus on the positives. I consoled myself with the knowledge that I was bettering myself and that things could have been much worse. I learned that it is important to be thankful in all things; no matter how dim the light, the light is still shining. I was still breathing and I had another day to do better. So I kept moving forward, I kept overcoming.

CHAPTER 11

THE MASQUERS CLUB: HOLLYWOOD LIFE

It was 1983 and I was homeless. The Masquers Club was there for me. The Masquers Club was organized to be a private place for the male movie stars to go relax, have fun, fellowship and also to discuss creative projects and other ventures. This four story mansion was right off of Hollywood Boulevard and North Sycamore. It was close to the Gremlin Chinese Theater and Magic Castle, which rest in the hills. This is where all the Magicians went to perform and be discovered. The Masquers Club had every amenity that you could think of: a dining room, a full Theater where the Hollywood A-List Actors would put on shows, and also a downstairs tavern with a hand carved bar. In the tavern, there was a stage where entertainers performed, socialized, and had drinks.

After 6pm, females were allowed to come to the club, but they had to be escorted by a male member of the club. It was not until after the 1970's that females were allowed in without a male member. A few years later, they then allowed females to join the club, but they had to be recommended by a male member.

Everybody who was anybody came through the Masquers Club at some point in time. Bob Duggan, who was the manager of the club at that time, invited me to join upon the introduction of one of my make up teachers who said it would be a great place for me to get experience in my field. Bob and I hit it off right away and he made me feel right at home. One day I took my friend Joseph, who had helped me years ago, to the club and he paid my dues to join.

The relationships that I built through membership in the Masquers club paid off. Being a member there allowed me to work on my craft, doing make up for many of their shows, and I also worked with lighting, staging and props during my time there. I gained both backstage and onstage experience as an actress in the plays they produced. I really learned a lot about theater and art production, and I got to network with the stars. More importantly, it gave me a place to stay when I was homeless. This was a mansion to the stars of stars.

Not too long after I joined the Masquers Club, it merged with another organization, The Variety Arts Club led by then-President actor and comedian Milton Berle. The two organizations merged to further their mutual creative arts goals and initiatives. Their first joint event was the roasting of Jim Baker, an editor for the *Los Angeles Times*. He wrote about the lives of the rich and famous, and all the stars came out. This was an elegant black tie event and it was huge in Hollywood. Everyone of importance was there and the paparazzi were all over the place to capture every moment.

I had the pleasure of attending the roast and met Milton Berle, Danny Thomas, Cesar Romero, the comic duo of Dan Rowan and Dick Martin, Sugar Ray

Robinson, Wilt Chamberlain, Benjamin Sherman "Scatman" Crothers who played in "Chico & The Man," and many others who came through on a regular basis. As I think back, I felt blessed to be in the midst of so many superstars in the 1980's. I was very comfortable being around all of these celebrities. I had gotten accustomed to being around them and even getting to know many of them personally during my time at The Masquers Club. I felt right at home among the stars; they were all very accepting of me and I really enjoyed being in such a creatively progressive environment. I was so inspired that I got back into playing the piano. I was going to City College and would get out and go to the club to hang out and practice my music.

There was always something going on there that was exciting and larger than life, and I was able to escape from the reality that I was homeless. They definitely kept me busy working on many major theater shows and I appreciate it because I learned so much from the best of the best in Hollywood. When I joined The Masquers Club, Anthony Caruso was the president or Harlequin. I am forever indebted to the wonderful people of this organization, and list the leaders in tribute: Robert Edeson, Douglas MacLean, Milton Sills, Sam Hardy, Mitchell Lewis, Antonio Lewis, Antonio Moreno, Joe E. Brown, Lowell Sherman, Frank Morgan, Pat O'Brien, Charles Chase, William Collier Sr., William B. Davidson, Robert Armstrong, Alan Mowbray, Lou Costello. Edward Arnold, Charles Coburn, Fred Niblo, Charles Kemper, Ralph Murphy, Fred Clark, Rhys Williams, Gene Autry, Frank Faylen, Harry Joe Brown, Allan Hersholt, Joseph Pasternak, Louis R. Lauria, and Pat Buttram.

CHAPTER 12

WITH GOD, ALL THINGS ARE POSSIBLE

I had to overcome various levels of internal obstacles that were trying the block me from my destiny that included a painful childhood, heartbreaking relationships, tragedy, deception, and fraud. Through hard work, dedication, faith in God and getting back up after being knocked down several times, I am now a highly sought after Entertainment Makeup Artist who works with A-List celebrities. It simply amazes me that I was among the trailblazers in beauty product innovation as well as in entrepreneurship during this time in our country's history. I am even more amazed by the experiences I continue to enjoy with God's blessings.

At a young age during a time where black people were not able to get a decent job, I was afforded the opportunity to dibble and dabble in the film industry doing background work. This time actually ignited my passion to later focus my talents in the film and entertainment arena. I worked on the film *Black Belt Jones* with Jim Kelly, a Karate movie, *Uptown Saturday Night* with Bill Cosby and Sidney Poitier, and also *Lets Do It Again* that starred Jimmy Walker and John Amos in addition to Cosby and Poitier. I worked with John Travolta, Martin Sheen, and so many other A-List Actors. Sammy Davis, Jr. actually helped me to celebrate my birthday one year at Lake Tahoe at the Sahara Club. He dedicated his show to me and had one of the waiters bring me champagne. He noticed they bought me domestic, and called out the entire wait staff saying, "You guys don't think we know anything about French Champagne? Bring my sister out some French Champagne." They did, by bringing out the biggest bottle of Dom Perignon they had. Sammy came over and personally toasted me and my friends during his show. When the show was over, he wished me a happy birthday again. I have had so many encounters both personally and professionally with the world's greatest entertainers.

Although I had experience in cosmetics and marketing beauty products, I did not necessarily have experience in the application of them, especially for the film industry. So I used my time on those sets to learn as much as I could by observing and asking lots of questions to those makeup artists who were working on the set. These opportunities excited me and made me realize that I definitely loved working in the film industry and desired to use my gifts and talents in makeup artistry for the long haul. Since then, I've had the honor to work on countless feature films like *The Walking Dead*, *Watson Goes to Birmingham*, *Barbershop 3* with Ice Cube, Cedric The Entertainer, Nicki Minaj, Common, Anthony Anderson and a host of other amazing actors; *Ride Along 2* with Ice Cube, Kevin Hart and so many others. *Bessie* was another, with Queen Latifah, Mo'Nique and Mike Epps. The Makeup Department Head for *Bessie* was nominated for a Primetime Emmy Award, and she named each member of the team - self included - in her press releases about this huge accomplishment.

I have mentioned that I have worked extensively with the Entertainment Mogul,

Tyler Perry, on his TV productions that include *For Better or Worse*, *Meet The Browns*, *House of Payne* and *Love thy Neighbor*. I worked on his movie, *For Colored Girls*, starring Kimberly Elise, Whoopi Goldberg, Anika Noni Rose, and a host of other great actresses. I worked on the 2012 television remake of *Steel Magnolias*, with Queen Latifah, Phylicia Rashad, Jill Scott, Condola Rashad, Alfre Woodard and many other esteemed Black actresses. I also worked on the television production of the "Red Bed Society," Series 1. I so enjoyed working on *Joyful Noise* with Kirk Franklin, Dolly Parton, Queen Latifah, Ke Ke Palmer, Courtney B. Vance, Jessie Martin and so many other talented entertainers. Most recently I worked on Marvel's *Bigfoot AKA Ant-Man* with Paul Rudd and Michael Douglas, *A Meyers Christmas*, Tupac's biopic *All Eyez On Me* directed by Benny Boom, and an Untitled Lee Daniels Pilot.

The fact that I have accomplished all these things shows that again, with God all things are possible and that perseverance pays off. I am thankful that I never gave up! When something is for you, it is for you and no obstacle, challenge, or adversity will be able to stop it unless you allow it. Make a decision today that you will not give up and that pursuing your passion, going after your destiny is your ultimate goal in life. You have to believe in yourself even when others do not. Cheer yourself on when others "boo" you. Make the decision to follow your dreams wholeheartedly. When backed with faith in God and a strong commitment to your cause, you will not fail. Remember, with God, ALL THINGS ARE POSSIBLE.

CHAPTER 13

MY LIFE'S MISSION

We all have a mission. We were put here on Earth to complete a specific mission from God. The mission is to help others to connect with God. We are here to save souls, it is all about Christ.

How do you know you are tasked for a specific mission? First, you must know God and have a relationship with Him. This relationship ensures that you know Him and that He knows you. You were not placed here to gather up material things and live haphazardly. You were sent here to know God and make Him known in the world. This is your - all of our - true mission in life. Regardless of what we go through in life, we must not be distracted from that mission. When we fall down, we must get back up and keep going. We must complete the assignments that our Creator sent us to Earth to complete.

This revelation led me to my next major assignment: one that gives hope and unites people. After visiting a local ministry with a friend, an Evangelist and her business partner, my eyes were opened to not only the need of more outreach programs for young people, but my call to action in this area.

While en route to a youth event that was organized by my friend, I saw so many unmet needs within our community. I heard a cry for help among the needy and underprivileged. When I arrived to the event, I was so inspired when I saw that the young people were being assisted. They received food, and were given positive role models who were speaking life into them and encouraging them to overcome various obstacles in the urban community such as gang violence, fatherless homes, and sexual violations. Being abandoned at a young age, some of these kids had kids of their own and had no clue as to how to take care of them. I saw the tremendous need for more people to step up to the plate and help to make positive changes within our community, with our kids who are the future.

While in this beautiful youth ministry service, I saw young people's lives being changed for the better by caring people who were definitely being used by God to deliver them from bondage and oppression. I saw hope restored and support being provided to people who had been left to fend for themselves. Those kids received much needed guidance and love. I saw the outreach coordinators meeting both the natural and Spiritual needs of humanity.

I was moved.

God gave me the vision to start a non-profit organization called UNITED WE STAND. I felt that if we all come together as a community, we can solve many of our community issues. We can do more together than apart, everyone doing their part, but collaborating to create a more impacting change. I believe in the motto "united we stand, divided we fall."

We cannot be selfish with our blessings. We have an obligation to share and meet the needs of others. If I see a need, I fill it if it is in my power to do so. If my brother is hungry, I feed him. No man is an island; we will all need someone at some time, so we should all be more open to meeting the needs of others. What you sow, you will reap. This is a biblical principle according to Galatians 6:9 in the Bible which states, "Don't be deceived, God is not mocked, whatever you sow, that shall you also reap." If you sow love, you will reap love, if you sow money, you will reap money, if you sow to meet someone's need, you will reap that in your time of need.

It is not rocket science that we can do more together and much change can be created through unity. That is how real lasting change occurs: through the actions of many people on one accord, working in unity towards a common goal. Significant global change rarely happens through the actions of one person alone. If we stand united, we could be a powerful force. My organization is dedicated to teaching young people their true potential in Christ and connecting them to resources that would help them become self sufficient and successful. What a blessing!

The tests and trials of life actually make you stronger and build your character. Although it hurts when you are going through them, the end results of your testing period are wisdom, strength and a resilience that will help you in fulfilling your purpose. Embrace your testing period and even celebrate it! A scripture that sums this concept up perfectly is Romans 8:28, "All things work together for the good of those who love the Lord and are called according to His purpose." Trust in that promise from the Lord knowing that when you are doing His will, and not doing your own thing, He will take care of you and everything will eventually work out.

CHAPTER 14

YOU CAN DO IT!

When I initially left home and was trying to figure out what I was going to do with my life, I went out looking for work and people asked me, "What can you do?" and I thought to myself, "I can't do anything." So I worked in factories or at restaurants bussing tables, doing hard work for little pay, because that is all I thought I could do. But one day I said to the Lord, "Lord, it just has to be more to me than this. Show me something that I can do." Then I set out to get a trade. Once I started looking within myself and took assessment of my needs and strengths, I was able to start working on me and finding things that I could do well and be paid well for them.

The take away is this: you may not know what you can do well, but you have to start doing something until you can find your passion or whatever comes natural to you. Do what you can do, what feels natural, or the things that you may have possibly done in the past, and always be open to learning more. This is exactly what I did and by doing so, I found my passions and began to live my dreams. Once I started accomplishing one goal, I started feeling good about myself. I was making it happen for myself - with God's direction of course - and I surprised myself doing so many new and exciting things. This encouraged me to do more. I felt unstoppable. Each time I would try something new and master it, I was motivated to try something else and master that. That is a part of growing and evolving. I am where I am because I was not afraid to try new things and go after what I felt belonged to me.

Although I heard lots of negative words spoken over me and was told how limited I was as a young black female with literacy challenges, I never bought into it. Deep in my heart I always knew that it was more to me than what others said about me. The more you believe in yourself, the stronger you get. The key is, you must believe in yourself before expecting others to do so.

I recall the times early in life when I did things for the approval of others. A lot of those times I allowed myself to be used for their good, not mine. I was holding on to dead weight and holding on to guys who were no good for me. I was almost 40 years old when I realized that I had wasted so much time doing things I was not happy with just to make others happy. The major lesson learned from all of my relationships, whether romantic or platonic, was that I could no longer allow myself to be used. I had to love myself and come to know that God lives in me.

You have greatness in you and you do not have to be anybody's doormat. Always feel good about yourself and who God created you to be. You do not have to be a fool to get someone to like you. That is what people with low self esteem do: they do things just to please others instead of doing what they know is best for themselves. Just like in my case, I developed low self esteem during my childhood and carried it right into my adult self. Lots of times, when I made poor choices because of my low self esteem, I threw a pity party and felt like "woe is me." I quickly learned that people do not care about your pity party. They are happy to see you down and out, feeling pitiful because then it is easier for them to use and manipulate you.

We have to teach others how to treat us by how we treat ourselves. When we have high self esteem and treat ourselves well, we will not allow others to treat us any type of way. Demand respect and those who do not give it are easily released from our lives.

It took me nearly forty years to learn these valuable lessons, but thank God that I have! I learned to value myself, to have self-respect and my life is all the better because of it.

CHAPTER 15

I AM A SUCCESS STORY

I stepped out on faith when I was in LA and started putting together my own beauty product line called Le Sure Dupre'. In 1988, I brought my line to Birmingham where I introduced it during my class reunion. I had actually created, developed and launched my very own cosmetic line! The Fairfield Industrial High School Reunion Committee assisted me with my launch of A Touch of Class with Pizzazz. They provided me with a venue, food, and promotion for the event. I was responsible for getting the talent, fashion and entertainment to make this event a success.

It was successful in terms of branding the name of my new business, but I fell short a bit in my marketing plan which should have focused on product purchases. I had no sales crew. People came from all over the country to attend; they learned about my new company and took this information back to their prospective states to promote. The lesson in this for business people and aspiring entrepreneurs is that you must have a strong marketing plan in place when launching a new product or business. Although I was happy with the promotion, which is always a good thing, I lost a lot of money that was not recouped in product sales.

I needed to regroup, so I put my company development on the back burner for a while to make money. A business opportunity arose for me to do a joint restaurant venture with my sister. We opened a restaurant and called it The Snack Bar in Birmingham. I put up all of the investment capital to start, bought all the supplies needed to open and right before we were scheduled to open, my sister decided to go in another direction and took a job. I was extremely let down and hurt because I never intended to run this business by myself. I did everything: I was the cook, the cleaner, the server, and any and everything else that was needed. I had help with bookkeeping though, thank God. It was very difficult, tiring, and I was being consumed in areas that I never signed up for. The business was doing pretty well, and picked up over the year that I worked it, but I did not like being alone in this huge endeavor. I was opening and closing alone, had to carry a gun late at night and was uncomfortable after having a few break-in attempts.

At one point, I had so many customers in the Fairfield community I could not keep up with the volume. We were beginning to be known and people seemed to love our fish and chicken. However, I walked away from the business because I felt I was working hard outside of my areas of skill and primary training. The reason that I actually got into the restaurant business was to help my sister who was a great cook and I felt that she had the skills to open her own business instead of working for others. I thought that I would be in a support role and assist with the business development of the restaurant, but still have the time to continue to focus on furthering my career in the beauty industry.

Owning and operating the restaurant was too much for one person. The cooking, cleaning, shopping and handling customer service issues got to be overwhelming to say the least, and I was completely stressed out most of the time. I got tired of smelling like fish and chicken all of the time, and closed the business. I needed a change, and when I was ready, I made it.

CHAPTER 16

I KNEW I COULD DO IT

After I closed the restaurant, I had a divine moment: I was in my kitchen and heard a commercial for a stage play called *Stop the Noise, Bring Back the Music* by Delilah Williams. I took down the information and readily prepared for the interview. Upon arriving at the interview, I felt really good as I was a professionally trained Makeup Artist in Alabama. Honestly, at that time there were very few, if any, who had gone to school for this trade. The main training schools were in New York, Florida, and California. I had a strong professional training history in the industry in California, working with the best of the best in niche areas such as special effects. I have to say that I was a rare jewel from this aspect and I was definitely qualified for this amazing opportunity. I was hired on the spot and it was on again! I was back traveling the world doing what I loved: working in theater. This was a new beginning for me.

Delilah wrote many plays, such as *Your Arms Are Too Short to Box with God, Somebody Ought to Tell God Thank You, Things Ain't What They Use To Be*, and as mentioned earlier, *Stop the Noise, Bring Back the Music*, plus many others. I traveled around the country working with the last two plays and made my home in Atlanta, Georgia.

I was blessed to be an entrepreneur; it felt great working for *me*. I was even more blessed that God maintained me through it all. I only have one regret: I wish I had known a little more about the business industry, though I did okay off of the little that I did know.

There is a lot to lose in business if you do not know about the ins and outs, and it can be very costly. Business politics is something that constantly comes up to battle you in business. I got kicked out of a business I was running in the mall because of business politics. A lot of times, people do not want you to be successful and that was the case in this particular situation. Previously, I was working at a very popular salon doing makeup and eyebrow arching. We would do makeovers, but we did not have a full line of makeup we used. One day I asked the owner if I could bring in my line of cosmetics (I told her that I had my own line). She told me that it would be great and that I could bring it in. So the next day I took it in. When I showed it to the owner she looked very surprised when she saw my line. She complimented me on how nice everything looked and how professionally it was put together, and then she told me that they did not have space for me to put it. She told me that I needed to get my own kiosk. I secured a contract with the mall manager for a kiosk under the agreement that I would do makeup and brow arching.

Soon after, the manager came back and told me I needed to sign a new agreement. This one prohibited me from arching eyebrows, it only allowed me to do cosmetic sells and makeovers. I knew this new change was because of the salon owner whose salon was also in the mall. I was doing very well for myself and I continued to arch eyebrows. The manager was not happy with me arching eyebrows, but did not say anything. Months later, the business picked up so much that I had to hire additional staff to manage our clientele. We had lines throughout the mall for our services and this caught the attention of the salon owner and the mall manager. He came to me and told me that I could not have another staff person working with me and that he only wanted one person working at a time. I responded by telling him that I am paying rent for a certain amount of space and that I should be able to hire whomever I need to work in my space. After that, he would not accept my rent; I was on a month to month lease and so he basically kicked me out of the mall without notice.

After I was kicked out of the mall, business dwindled as I tried to do work in other shops, but it just was not the same. Months later I ended up getting a space right across from the mall and business was doing really well, but the location was not ideal. Not to be outdone, I opened a full service salon with a nail tech and massage therapist. We offered facials, and we had a boutique with vintage clothing. We had a photography studio as well. My new business offered much more than the standard hair salon at this time. I invested so much money in the development of this location, however I chose poor contractors who really messed me over. They took my money and even stole from me. With all of the challenges to open and launch this new venture, I had a few friends who stuck it out with me and I was able to launch on time. I enjoyed the business and my customers, but I eventually yearned for more freedom and flexibility than having a shop would allow. So after my five year lease was up, I closed my business and started booth renting to focus more on my venture into the movie business doing make up. That was something I truly wanted to do, working with films, and I thanked God for the opportunity.

I am grateful for my early introduction to Tyler Perry while he was still getting his vision together. This allowed me to see up close and personal how his dream came to fruition. God gave him a big entrepreneurial vision as a writer, director, and stage play and film producer. He started out almost as a one man band with his stage plays, and now, not only have his stage plays become blockbuster hits, so have his movies!

Tyler Perry developed a multi-million dollar production company, Tyler Perry Studios, right here in Atlanta that now employs thousands of people. He had a vision and stuck with it despite how hard it was initially to get the ball rolling. Now we all see the magnificent fruits of his labor. Like me, he experienced a period of homelessness while trying to birth his vision, but he did not let that stop him from moving forward and pursuing his dream.

I remember going through a really hard time during my early days working in the film industry in Atlanta. I had been working with Tyler Perry Studios for a few years, and at the time that is where most of my work came from. Things changed in the makeup department when new department heads were hired. When this happened, a lot of the familiar faces disappeared and were replaced by friends of the new department head. My hours were cut to the point that I was basically not working. I happened to run into Tyler Perry in the hallway on Actors Row. I was in bad shape and needed to work. I broke down because no one was calling me anymore. I had no money, did not know where my next meal was coming from, and was at my lowest point. I was extremely emotional. I told him that I needed a job. He stopped everything, took me to the side, told me to dry my eyes, and that everything would be alright. He really helped me out right then and there, and gave me a job. I was so happy and surprised. I was crying and he hugged me then he said, "Go wipe your face clean because I don't want anybody thinking I'm over here beating you up." He immediately went into the makeup room and spoke to the department head and told him to hire me on full time hours.

What a blessing, and lifesaver, Mr. Perry has been to me! That act of kindness was enough to keep me floating from that day until now. His heart is so huge; he cares deeply for people and his staff. I know for a fact that no matter what, he will always be a blessed man because of how he pours out unselfishly to others. I believe his life and his seemingly "overnight success" is a testament to this: when you give to help meet the needs of others, God will always give back to you in abundance.

CHAPTER 17

WE ALL HAVE A STORY

Well, I knew I needed to write a book for a while now. My Pastor, Andre Landers, the shepherd of Higher Living Christian Church in Georgia, tells us that we all have books inside of us. I agree with him because we all have a story to tell, a message that can encourage someone else.

Encouraging youth is a passion of mine. When I see young people, I just want to talk to them and tell them how great they are. I realize that we must start early in that encouragement, while they are babies and toddlers, letting them know how great they are and what wonderful specimens God made them to be. We need to keep telling them that as often as possible while they are very young. We must try to find out what talents or interests children have and encourage them to pursue them. In order to do that, we have to spend time observing them and helping them find out their passions. We then have to nurture their dreams, instead of beating them up - emotionally, physically or verbally - when they seem slow to learn. It is not beneficial to pass judgment and keep pointing out their flaws. When I was a young child, I always wanted to encourage slow learners and tell them there was something they were good at because they also had greatness within. My father only had a first grade education and I was always in awe of all the things he could do. He fixed everything in our home, we never had anyone come over to repair anything. If the washing machine broke down, daddy would disassemble it and put it back together like new.

I kept on believing that there was greatness in me as well. I found myself doing much more professionally than people who were more educated than I. I have a secret: most people look at you through their eyes, their short comings, then they want to place those things on you. I am here to tell you that you do not have to accept anyone else's opinions about you or your abilities. Do not allow others to stigmatize you. You have to keep your eyes focused on your dreams and where you want to be, and meditate on that. Stop looking at what it is and imagine what could be if you have faith and work hard. I do not care what it is, just stay with it! We will all be all right if we just do that.

You take one step, God will take another one. Before you know it, the things that you had been waiting for will have already started to happen for you. Keep your eyes on the prize; that is how you overcome, you believe and you have faith and you keep your eyes on your goals instead of your circumstances.

Figure out exactly what it is that you are trying to accomplish. Start thinking about how you are going to accomplish it. You have to make a plan. Where do you want to be in two years? In five years? Think about how you will do it, then start working on it. God will open doors for you, and introduce you to those you need to meet in order to get to your place of destiny. I am a witness! You tell God what you want and He will make it happen, if you truly believe.

Do your footwork with your goals in mind and put your faith in action. Whatever it is you want to do, get as much training in that area as possible. Everything I have wanted to do in this life, I have done it. Writing this book and now speaking into the lives of people all over the world has been a dream come true, a goal long overdue, but I finally did it. Now I do not recommend that you wait as long as I did, but it does not matter what age you are, you can still pursue your dreams right where you are. There are no limitations as long as you are breathing. When I was a little girl I said, "I want to live in California," and I did. I said, "I want to live in New York," and I did that, too. So many things I said I wanted to do and places I wanted to go, and I did them in faith.

I remember another time when I saw the power of vision and positive confession at work in my life. I always noticed this particular boutique while walking to the supermarket, which was not far from my apartment. One day I said that I wanted to have a boutique just like that one. Little did I know that I would actually own that very boutique in the future! This is another example of the power of our words. The things that we think, say, and believe are the things that happen in our lives - whether good or bad.

When leaving LA to move back to Birmingham, I said that

• I did not want to live with anybody

• I did not want another apartment and

• I did not want a job where I had to work for someone else.

Subsequently, I got a house without having a job. I assumed the loan and all I had to do was keep the loan current for a year, then the Federal Housing Authority (FHA) transferred the loan into my name. No credit checks, no one asked me for my earning statements or anything. I got that house with no job because I wanted it, I spoke it into the atmosphere and I believed that I would get it. I left the rest to God and He came through for me.

There are so many things waiting on you. If you believe, they can happen for you too. This was not the only time this happened for me. My next house came to me basically the same way. I got into the house that I am currently living in by the grace and favor of God. I again had no credit checks or income verifications. When God is in the mist of something, it will work out as smooth as butter. Do not worry about anything, instead pray about everything, and the peace of God will come over you and cover you. Release the details of the *how* to God our Father and He is wise enough to work out every situation in your life with no problems. After all, He is God.

CHAPTER 18

WHATEVER *YOUR* "IT" IS, YOU WILL OVERCOME IT

If you allow it, the pain that you experience in life can propel you into your purpose, into doing the very thing that you were created to do.

It has been a tough road as a minority female from humble beginnings with educational limitations, but I made it. I accomplished my professional goals, was a trendsetter in the entrepreneurial world, entertainment industry, and also a major part of history during a very tumultuous time in the United States. In 1963, I was involved in the Civil Rights Movement. I went to jail for fighting for the next generation. It hurts my heart that despite how much we have done, the Movement came at a time when it was hard for me to get work in a field that I pioneered.

There was so much going on during the Civil Rights Movement that it would take books and books to cover it all. Each day at 12pm, which was my lunch hour at school, I would walk over to 16th Street Baptist Church. It was one block from my school. At the church, we would meet and there would be different leaders that would speak to us, preparing us for the march that we were getting ready to do. They would tell us all the Do's and Don'ts, and kept reminding us that this was a non violent movement. We were told that if we could not adhere to the non violent approach, then we should not participate in the march. They organized groups to be in certain areas. People were to the north, south, east and west, making it difficult for the police because they would have to spread out because they did not know where the protest was going to be.

In Birmingham, all of the Civil Rights leaders stayed at the A.G. Gaston Motel Lounge because it was the only decent place for black people to stay. Dr. Martin Luther King, Jr. and the other leaders would stay there during the week and go home on the weekend. Daily, there was a lot of work that we all had to do. The days would start with planning and organizing meetings at the church, we would then participate in scheduled protests, marches and sit ins, then we would take a break around 3pm. I would go home, have dinner, then clean up and change clothes to go back downtown to the mass meeting at the 16th Street Baptist Church which was one block over from the A.G. Gaston Motel Lounge. The evening meetings would usually be led by Dr. King, Minister Ralph Abernathy, or a guest speaker like Rev. Fred Shuttlesworth. There was usually standing room only, especially if Dr. King was speaking, so if you wanted to get a seat, you had to get there very early.

Rev. Shuttlesworth was the person who actually brought Dr. King and the Civil Rights Movement to Birmingham. We often gathered in Kelly Ingram Park, since it was across the street from the church and often the crowd was so massive that the church could not hold everyone. This was also the historic location where the police officers let their dogs loose on the protestors. It did not matter if they were young or old or babies, the police let their dogs attack the peaceful protesters without any regrets. At the same time, the firefighters would hose us down. We would have to run and hide as best we could behind cars and trees to prevent our skin from being torn off due to the power of the water that came from their hoses. They were sinister in their attacks: they would allow us to protest, sit in, and march in the downtown business district; the police and fireman would just follow us as we marched peacefully. But as soon as we got into the black business district on Fourth Avenue around the park, all hell would break loose. That is when they would let the dogs go and spray us with the hoses for no reason.

When you visit this historic park now, you can see the statues of dogs being let loose on young children. I, along with many other young people, went to jail for standing up for what we believed in: justice and liberty. It was the young people, generally ages 9 to 25, who actually led the movement and made a difference as the older people had to go to work and make a living for their families. We, as youth, were able to sacrifice and go to jail on behalf of our people.

One time a black man saved me from being attacked by a police dog. The police officer was holding onto the dog as he was putting him on me but holding the dog just enough that he did not bite me; I just stood still because I was afraid. Then that black man came out of nowhere and just started stabbing the dog. The policemen started running over and jumped on him, they beat him and carried him to jail. I saw some of the most horrific injustices ever at the hands of police officers; they had no mercy on the elderly or the feeble. It was a regular sight to see the officers dragging 60 and 70 year old women down the street like animals; exposing all of their private parts. I am thankful to God that I was never seriously hurt during the protests.

I actually went to jail twice, one week each time. The first time, I was arrested with Dr. King on Good Friday and I stayed in jail until the following Saturday. The conditions in the jails were deplorable to say the least. In reflection, it is incredible to me that I actually shared a jail cell with the iconic leader before they separated the males from the females. While we were in jail together, he wrote the famous "Letter from the Birmingham Jail." I remember Dr. King voicing how he saw something special about me, how I was called to impact the world with my future gifts and talents. The police officers called out names to separate the men from the women to take us to our cells. When they called out my name "Veronica Lake Cox," Dr. King commented and said to me, "With a famous name like that you gotta do something with it." I replied, "I am, I'm here with you!" We both laughed. He responded, "Well, that's a start." Neither one of us had ANY IDEA how famous he would be, how important our activism, leadership, and courageous actions would be to the United States and the world.

I recall after one of the mass meetings my sister, cousin, and I went to the AG Gaston Motel Lounge. Dr. King and Rev. Abernathy were sitting at the table and invited us to join them. A radio DJ known as "Tall Paul" was also at the table. He worked for WENN Radio Station. Dr. King asked "Tall Paul" whom I was acquainted with to go to WENN Radio Station, which was a block away, to bring back the news updates. This station would air news to the world about what was going on with the movement, specifically the leaders. Paul asked me to come with him to the station and I did. One day I was going to the drug store and ran into Dr. King. He was alone. I spoke to him and he stopped and we talked for a short while. I asked for his autograph. I said, "Dr. King, may I have your autograph because one day you might be famous," he just laughed and gave it to me.

I was honored to have met and served with Dr. Martin Luther King, Jr. I am only scratching the surface in sharing with you a few of the things that I experienced during the Movement. I hope that young people today and future generations appreciate the sacrifices that the older generations made so that they can enjoy the lives that they live today and beyond. Because of the blood, sweat, and tears of our folks involved in the Movement, our young people are able to attend integrated schools and get a quality education, eat where they want, vote, and enjoy basic civil liberties. It hurts my heart when young people look down on the elderly or disrespect them, disregarding the sacrifices that the elderly made for them to experience the freedom that they have today.

I am still fighting, I'm still overcoming. There are still other milestones I want to reach. I am still "climbing that mountain," and fearlessly jumping off of it too, by challenging myself at every stage in my life.

Once you believe you can do one thing and accomplish it, you move on to something bigger and accomplish that. Before, I would do things looking to please others. I am a giver by nature, so it is always in my heart to help others succeed in life. If there is something in my power that I can do for someone I care about, I will because I want them to win. I came to realize that my own goals, visions, and dreams were worth fighting for.

If you are alive and breathing and believing in yourself, you will overcome anything. I say that with extreme confidence. With God inside of you giving Divine assistance, there is nothing that you cannot overcome. He already has your destiny planned out, all you have to do is believe and push forward and walk in faith!

If you believe you will overcome, you will overcome. No one ever stays in the same place: you are either going forward or you are going backwards - you are not standing still. By moving forward, you will inevitably overcome. Keep taking one step at a time. There is a popular saying that goes, "It's hard by the yard, but it's a cinch by the inch." That means if you take a little step at a time, it is easier than trying to take huge steps all at once. Each day, focus on taking one little step. Keep your goal in your mind. Do not lose hope! Have faith in yourself and know that you *will* get to where you want to go in life. It all starts in your mind with the thoughts that you think. Everything starts as a thought. Whatever you think is what you will manifest. Proverbs 23:7 says, "As a man (or woman) thinks in his (or her) heart, so is he (or she)." So, the main way to overcome in life is by overcoming negative thoughts.

Let this be your daily meditation:

"I WILL OVERCOME, I WILL OVERCOME.

WHATEVER LIFE'S CHALLENGES ARE, I WILL OVERCOME IT!

BECAUSE GREATER IS HE THAT IS IN ME, THAN HE THAT IS IN THE WORLD."

I will continue to overcome all that comes my way, no matter what "it" is because greatness is in me.

1 John 4:4 "Ye are of God, little children, and have overcome them: because greater is He that is in you, than he that is in the world."

Forgiveness

I am so thankful for the gift of a loving and forgiving spirit. Forgiveness is so important to our daily growth. In order for us to move forward in life we must forgive each other. We cannot afford to let the fuss of hurt and pain that has been afflicted on us by others block our joy and success in life. We must look at them as growing pains because it helps us to become stronger people.

After each instance of pain in my life, I became mentally and emotionally stronger, and stronger in my self-belief. I had to forgive in order to grow, as I could not carry the baggage of someone else's hurt and pain. I learned that hurt people, hurt people because they have not forgiven themselves nor have they forgiven others.

We must always forgive, no matter what has been done to you (or what you think has been done to you). Forgiveness frees you to love more and to be more of what God wants you to be. In order to see God you must have a forgiving heart.

We must pray for people who are hurting, pray that they will find peace and joy before it is too late. I forgive each and every person who played a part in the hurt and pain I experienced in my life. If it had not been for those people and the part they played in my life, I would not be the person I am today: strong, mature, motivated, aggressive, determined and successful. So I just want to say from the bottom up my heart thank you! Thank you! I love you all.

About the Author

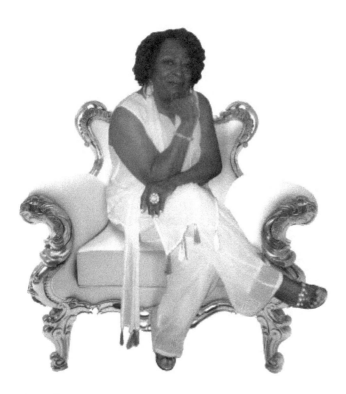

Veronica Cox is an extraordinary woman who teaches others to conquer the mountains in their lives. Veronica is a wildly successful makeup artist who has worked on several big-budget films and Emmy Award winning television shows; creator of her own makeup line; founder of a non-profit to help children; and Civil Rights pioneer, a "Foot Solider for Freedom" who marched with Dr. King. But she had to face and overcome incredible personal and professional obstacles to reach that success - abuse, betrayal, and loss - and now shares the wisdom and strength gained during those times to empower others.

Veronica's struggles began early with the rejection of her mother, and did not get any easier - she was jilted at the altar, betrayed by her business partner, and lost her best friend to suicide. All the while, she worked to create the life she wanted, embracing her skills and talents as a stylish and savvy entrepreneur in fashion, beauty, and retail. With each trial, Veronica's faith in herself and trust in God's perfect will in her life grew... And she realized that the knowledge that she gleaned from each experience was not only hers to enjoy, but was to be shared with others to conquer their fears and trepidation, and find their purpose in the world!

"All things are possible with faith. With faith, we know before we even see the mountain of challenge that we will conquer it and be left stronger because of it."